PARKINSON'S

One Step at a Time

Problems and Answers
For Patients and Health Professionals

Third Edition

J. David Grimes, MD • David A. Grimes, MD

PARKINSON'S
SOCIETY OF
OTTAWA-
CARLETON

Published by:

Parkinson's Society of Ottawa-Carleton
1053 Carling Avenue
Ottawa, Ontario
Canada K1Y 4E9

Canadian Cataloguing in Publication Data

Grimes, J. David, 1939 – Parkinson's: One Step at a Time:
Problems and Answers for Patients and Health Professionals

3rd ed.
Includes index
ISBN 0-9694243-1-0

    1.Parkinson's disease – Treatment

    2. Parkinson's disease – Treatment – Popular works.

    I. Grimes, David A., 1966-

    II. Parkinson's Society of Ottawa-Carleton.

    III. Title.

RC382.G75 1999   616.8'3306   C99-901364-5

Dedication and Personal Note

To Sharon Grimes, my wife, partner and caregiver who has shepherded me through my illness over the past 15 years. The rare immune lung disorder that began in 1986 resulted in a double lung transplant in 1991 and the required anti-rejection drugs led to the development of successfully treated Hodgkin's disease in 1995. Like Parkinson's, these illnesses result in problems in almost all parts of one's body and Sharon has handled each setback with optimism, encouragement and love.

Mark Twain said "Write what you know about" and I certainly feel qualified to write from the viewpoint of a patient. I have experienced many of the problems discussed in the book and given suggestions and tips that benefited me.

The special relationship between the patient and doctor is crucial and I usually experienced warm compassion and encouragement but also met physicians who were blunt, cold and upsetting. It is so nice on a bad day to hear things from your doctor like "we will work this out together"; " I have seen this before and it will settle", and the question we all long for at the end of a visit, "is there anything else you want to discuss."

I am a great believer in optimism, living with your illness and its limitations, and getting on with life. I was able to return to work after each of my major illnesses but by December 1997 it seemed appropriate to retire. Our son David has taken over as Director of the Parkinson's clinic at the Ottawa Hospital and what a wonderful joy this is for his father and mother.

J. David Grimes

Preface to the Third Edition

New knowledge about all aspects of Parkinson's and its' management is developing at a rapid pace. This third edition of One Step at a Time has been completely revised, expanded and contains a wealth of new information with many new sections. It is a comprehensive handbook that explains everything that patients, their families and health professionals need to know about Parkinson's. Reviews of research, new therapies and potential future treatments are included. New and innovative approaches to surgical treatment are detailed. New theories on the cause are outlined and new knowledge of the molecular genetics of Parkinson's is presented. Sixty percent of the book is devoted to practical and useful tips for the common problems of the disease. These are the small things that can, if recognized and treated, make a big difference to the comfort of the patient. There are new facts on memory, sleep disorders, bowel and bladder dysfunction, sexual problems, fractures and osteoporosis, surgery and in hospital care, estrogen, pregnancy, alternative medicine, coping with the disease and care at the end of life.

As with previous editions we have presented the book with a "patient first" attitude and a tone of optimism, hope and compassion. The book addresses the "whole patient" and all of the large and small nuisance problems that may affect almost every body system over the course of an illness that often spans 30 or more years. The goal of every medical visit should be **to get the little things right**. A World Charter of Rights for people with Parkinson's has been developed and contains the following points that we firmly agree with: referral to a doctor with a special interest in Parkinson's; to receive an accurate diagnosis; to have access to support services; to receive continuous care and to take part in managing your illness.

Preparation and research for this third edition began as the second was finished and consisted of the collection and review of more than 1000 articles, attendance at scientific meetings, discussion with colleagues and most importantly, working with patients. Since the last edition a number of new drugs have become available to treat the many components of Parkinson's. As we better understand the biochemistry of the brain, there have been major advances in our understanding and treatment of emotional and memory problems, and sleep disturbances.

Susan Ziebarth and Ken Gorman of the Parkinson's Society of Ottawa-Carleton gave support and advice as did Keith Christopher and Grant Walsh of the Board of Directors.

Kelly Grimes Ohman coordinated the project, edited the manuscript and set the pace for timely completion. She and her husband Hans did the table of contents and index and Kelly altered sentences that were too long and contained too much "doctor speak." Kristen Grimes performed a multitude of tasks over the past many years to keep our files and new information current and readily available.

J. David Grimes

David A. Grimes
September 1999

The Authors:

J.DAVID GRIMES, MD, FRCPC

Dr. Grimes was Director of the Parkinson's Clinic at the Ottawa Hospital from 1977 to 1997. When he retired for health reasons he was Chief Executive Officer of the Loeb Health Research Institute, Senior Vice-President Research and Academic Affairs at the Ottawa Civic Hospital, a member of the Parkinson's Study Group and Professor of Medicine (Neurology), University of Ottawa. He continues as: Medical Advisor to the Parkinson's Society of Ottawa-Carleton, a member of the Board of Directors and Executive committee of the Loeb Health Research Institute, a member of the Civic Foundation and emeritus Professor of Medicine (Neurology) University of Ottawa. Dr. Grimes has written extensively on Parkinson's and has authored numerous scientific publications and teaching and review articles.

DAVID A. GRIMES, MD, FRCPC

Dr. Grimes is Director of the Parkinson's Disease Centre and Movement Disorders Clinic at the Ottawa Hospital. He has recently completed a combined fellowship in molecular genetics at the Centre for Neurodegenerative Diseases in Toronto and in clinical movement disorders at the Morton and Gloria Shulman Movement Disorder Centre at the Toronto Hospital. His laboratory research program involves the identification of new genes involved in a wide variety of movement disorders including Parkinson's disease. He will be involved in the surgical treatment program for Parkinson's.

In Appreciation

Peggy Gray has been the nurse coordinator of the Parkinson's Clinic at the Ottawa Hospital for 20 years. She has cared for our patients with skill, love and compassion. Peggy and her husband Doug participated in the first two editions of **One Step at a Time** and Doug, a skilled author, wrote the conclusion for the second edition. Doug died in June 1999 and the conclusion to the third edition remains as Doug wrote it five years ago.

Contents

CHAPTER 1: OVERVIEW OF PARKINSON'S 1

SYMPTOMS 1

   Tremor 1

   Rigidity 2

   Bradykinesia 2

   Postural Instability 3

SCALES FOR RATING DISABILITY 4

   Hoehn and Yahr 4

   Schwab and England Scale 5

INCIDENCE AND PROGNOSIS 6

CAUSE 7

GENETICS 9

ENVIRONMENTAL TOXIN EXPOSURE 12

YOUNG-ONSET PARKINSON'S 13

BRAIN SCANS 15

TYPES OF PARKINSONISM AND DISORDERS

WHICH MAY BE CONFUSED WITH PARKINSON'S 16

   Classical Parkinson's disease 17

   Essential Tremor 17

   Drug Induced Parkinsonism 19

   Atypical Parkinsonism or Parkinson's Plus 21

VERY EARLY SYMPTOMS OF PARKINSON'S 26

CHAPTER 2: CURRENT DRUG THERAPIES 27

LEVODOPA AND ITS COMPLICATIONS 29

    Is levodopa toxic? 29

    Daily Mobility Fluctuations 35

    "On-Off" Phenomenon 36

    End-Of-Dose Failure ("wearing off" effect) 36

    Freezing 37

    No "On" Response 38

    Less Common Fluctuations 38

    Involuntary Movements (Dyskinesias) 41

    Akathisia (Restlessness) 44

    When dyskinesias occur, your doctor may try
    the following: 44

DOPAMINE AGONISTS 45

COMT INHIBITORS 51

MONOAMINE OXIDASE-B (MAO-B) INHIBITORS
(SELEGILINE-DEPRENYL-ELDEPRYL) 53

AMANTADINE 56

ANTICHOLINERGICS 58

DOMPERIDONE 60

DRUGS FOR ESSENTIAL TREMOR
(PROPRANOLOL, PRIMIDONE) 61

LONG TERM DRUG ADJUSTMENTS
FOR PARKINSON'S 63

    Tips for Medication 63

OVER THE COUNTER DRUG WARNING 66

PARTICIPATION IN CLINICAL TRAILS 66

THE PLACEBO RESPONSE 67

ALTERNATIVE THERAPY .67

CHAPTER 3: CURRENT SURGICAL TREATMENTS 69

LESIONING PROCEDURES 71

DEEP BRAIN STIMULATION 73

CANDIDATES FOR SURGICAL PROCEDURES 76

CHAPTER 4: RESEARCH AND NEW THERAPIES 77

New Methods of Delivery 78

Methionine 79

Lysoganglioside 79

Gene Therapy 79

Neuroprotection 80

Glutamate Antagonists 81

Stem Cells 81

Growth Factors 82

Other Novel Therapies 83

Tissue Implantation 84

DISABILITY WITH ADVANCED PARKINSON'S 86

BRAIN TISSUE DONATION 87

CHAPTER 5: COMMON PROBLEMS AND TIPS TO OVERCOME THEM 89

HANDWRITING 89

MEMORY DISORDERS AND EMOTIONAL PROBLEMS . .89

Cognitive (Thinking) Impairment 90

Confusion and Hallucinations 94

Behavioural Impairments (Depression, Anxiety, Panic Attacks and Agitation) 100

SLEEP PROBLEMS 102

Insomnia 103

Increased Daytime Sleepiness 105

Upsets During Sleep 106

Sleep Benefit 107

Morning Worse 107

Restless Leg Syndrome .108

Leg Cramps 109

FATIGUE 110

BLADDER PROBLEMS 111

SEXUAL PROBLEMS 114

POSTURAL HYPOTENSION 118

THE DIGESTIVE SYSTEM .123

Drooling 125

Dry Mouth and Mouth Care Advice 126

Dental Care 127

Loss of Smell and Taste .128

Swallowing Difficulty .129

Impaired Gastric Emptying 134

Drug Related Nausea and Vomiting 136

Tips for Nausea and Vomiting 136

Constipation 137

Weight Loss, Nutrition and the Low Protein Diet 142

FRACTURES, OSTEOPOROSIS AND PREVENTION . . .146

SPEECH (DYSARTHRIA) 148

SKIN PROBLEMS AND CARE 152

Facial Skin 153

Eyelids 153

Dry Body Skin 154

Sweating Abnormalities 155

FOOT PAIN AND FOOT CARE 156

PAIN AND SENSORY SYMPTOMS 158

SHOULDER PAIN 161

LEG SWELLING (EDEMA) 161

SHORTNESS OF BREATH 163

VISUAL AND EYE PROBLEMS 164

DRIVING 166

ALCOHOL 168

GAIT 169

FALLS AND THEIR PREVENTION 177

EXERCISE AND PHYSIOTHERAPY 183

SCOLIOSIS 195

HAND DEFORMITY 197

HOSPITAL CARE INCLUDING SURGERY 197

HUMOUR 200

EMPLOYMENT 201

ESTROGEN 202

PREGNANCY 203

PATIENT SERVICES 206

Home Care 207

Meals on Wheels 207

Professional Homemaking Services 207

Day Hospital Programs .207

Respite Care Programs .208

Permanent Placement 208

Transportation Services .208

Parkinson's Associations 209

Directory of Resources for Senior Citizens 210

ASSISTIVE DEVICES AND TECHNIQUES 210

TRAVEL 213

COPING WITH THE ILLNESS 214

CARE AT THE END OF LIFE 222

CONCLUSION 223

INDEX **225**

APPENDIX: RECORD OF PERSONAL PARKINSON'S

HISTORY AND TREATMENT **231**

Chapter 1
Overview of Parkinson's

James Parkinson, who was a general practitioner in London England first described "the shaking palsy". His report was published in 1817 and contained the clinical symptoms of the disorder. Parkinson's is a progressive disorder of the central nervous system. A loss of dopamine in the brain occurs which causes **a set of four symptoms and signs: tremor, slowness, rigidity, bradykinesia (slow movements)** and loss of balance. Tremor and rigidity often occur initially on one side only.

Symptoms

Tremor

Tremor is a rhythmic involuntary movement which may affect the limbs, face or jaw. The most common tremor is a movement of the thumb and first finger giving a pill rolling effect. Tremor is caused by the alternating contraction of opposed muscle groups. This is the most bothersome of all the symptoms but is the least disabling. Parkinson's patients typically have a **resting tremor**, which means that the tremor ceases when reaching or performing some activity. Recordings made from the globus pallidus during pallidotomy reveal cells firing at the same rate as rest tremor. **Action tremor or tremor which occurs on movement**, may also accompany resting tremor but is not a typical part of the disorder (see section on Essential Tremor). Resting tremor is seen at some stage in most patients with classical Parkinson's but in some series up to 25% do not have rest tremor. It is infrequent in the other illnesses which mimic the disorder. Parkinson's patients who begin their illness with tremor tend to have a milder course with their illness. Some patients have a feeling of tremor inside their chest, abdomen or limbs but tremor is not seen (see sensory symptoms).

Rigidity

The muscular stiffness and increased muscle tone of rigidity is demonstrated by a resistance to passive movement of joints, for example the elbow, wrist and neck. Patients are usually not aware of rigidity but are more troubled with slowness. Rigidity is not as definite a symptom of parkinsonism as resting tremor and is more apparent to the examining doctor than to the patient.

Bradykinesia

This is **slowness of movement** and patients take longer to complete an activity. As well, the associated movements in undertaking an activity are reduced. For example, less arm swing when walking, not crossing the legs when sitting, slower facial movements, or reduced eye blinking which may result in a mask-like or staring expression. More time and effort may be needed to perform the normal activities of daily living. **Bradykinesia eventually becomes a much greater disability than tremor or rigidity**. The degree of bradykinesia correlates with the severity of dopamine neuron cell loss. It is tested by observing the slowness of a patient rising from a chair and slowness and difficulty in sustaining rapid finger-to-thumb movements with one or both hands. Levodopa is the best drug for bradykinesia.

After the disability has been present for some time, the normal walking pattern of the heel striking the floor first is reversed and a toe-first walk develops. Stride is reduced and a shuffling gait develops. Turning is slowed and the feet drag, causing noise. Some patients have brief halts and stalls termed "freezing" (see section on Fluctuations). Arm swing may be decreased and hand tremor may increase when walking.

Postural Instability

The progressive decline of postural reflexes **causing a loss of balance** is probably the most disabling of all parkinsonian symptoms. This becomes more prevalent as the illness progresses. Posture is stooped and the knees are flexed when walking. The patient may also develop a progressive lean to one side. Walking and turning are unsteady, and falls will occur. A patient if pushed slightly backwards when standing may fall straight back with no attempt to recover. This is because the ability to recover from minor losses of balance is diminished. This problem becomes less responsive to levodopa later in the illness but in typical Parkinson's some response is still seen. In other forms of parkinsonism, the balance response to levodopa is often very poor. Turning in bed is also more difficult later in the illness but it also retains some response to levodopa.

The presence of more one-sided signs and a good response to levodopa make the diagnosis of Parkinson's even more secure. It may take several years for symptoms to become more definite.

Scales For Rating Disability

There are many diverse and varied scales for determining disability. These tools of assessment include Hoehn and Yahr, the Unified Parkinson's Disease Rating Scale (UPDRS) and Schwab and England. UPDRS is a detailed and extensive scoring system and will not be outlined below. It evaluates more than 40 different aspects of Parkinson's, including depression, swallowing, dressing and gait. These scales are used by clinic nurses and neurologists to document changes.

Hoehn and Yahr

There are five stages of parkinsonian disability according to the Hoehn and Yahr scale:

Stage I

One-sided tremor or rigidity - with or without slowness of movement. Mildly affected patients at Stage I may not need any treatment but patients with moderate disability will be much more comfortable with therapy.

Stage II

Moderate tremor or rigidity occurring on both sides with bradykinesia. Symptoms will be improved with amantadine, levodopa or a dopamine agonist. The most common treatment is levodopa. The early use of dopamine agonists is being accepted as newer more potent drugs are developed.

Stage III

Significant tremor, rigidity and/or bradykinesia. This is accompanied by mobility problems. **Difficulties in postural**

control develop; there is unsteadiness on turns, and hesitations, halts and freezes when starting to walk. Patients begin to notice fluctuations in their level of function during a day and may experience dyskinesias (drug induced involuntary movements). The major new problem at this stage is balance difficulty.

Stage IV

More severe disability, but still able to walk. Bradykinesia is more severe and patients require some assistance with activities of daily living. If fluctuations are present they too will be more severe.

Stage V

Loss of ability to function independently. Postural defects are severe and independent mobility is impossible.

Note: Patients with severe mobility fluctuations may vary between stages I and V.

Schwab and England Scale

The Schwab and England is a scale used in assessing a patient's level of independence:

100% Completely independent. Able to do all chores without slowness, difficulty and impairment. Essentially normal. Unaware of any difficulty.

90% Completely independent. Able to do all chores with some degree of slowness, difficulty and impairment. Might take twice as long. Beginning to be aware of difficulty.

80% Completely independent in most chores. Takes twice as long. Conscious of difficulty and slowness.

70% Not completely independent. More difficulty with some chores. Three to four times as long in some. Must spend a large part of the day with chores.

60% Some dependency. Can do most chores, but exceedingly slowly and with much effort. Errors; some tasks impossible.

50% More dependent. Help with half of chores, shower, etc. Difficulty with everything.

40% Very dependent. Can assist with all chores, but few alone.

30% With effort, now and then does a few chores alone or begins alone. Much help needed.

20% Nothing alone. Can be a slight help with some chores. Severe invalid.

10% Totally dependent, helpless. Complete invalid.

Note: Patients with severe mobility fluctuations may vary greatly. For example a patient during a good or "on" period may function at 75%, yet when a bad or "off" period occurs they may revert to a 25% level of function. Not all patients experience all these stages.

Incidence and Prognosis

Parkinson's is one of the most common progressive neurological disorders, affecting as many as three percent of adults over the age of 65. It usually begins between the ages of 50 and 65 with an average age of onset of 60. It is much more prevalent in the 65 to 90 age group but five to ten percent of patients have symptoms before the age of 40 years (see section on Young-Onset). Parkinson's is slightly more common in men. **The outlook for Parkinson's patients improved markedly with the development of levodopa therapy** in the early 1970's. Patients who were previously confined to bed became mobile again. With modern drug therapy, **disability is reduced at all stages and mortality is decreased**. Unfortunately, there are no currently available therapies that have been shown to have a major impact on the progression of the disease. In the more advanced stage, disability is mainly due to **medication-related** problems (which can respond to drug changes) and **balance difficulties** (that do not respond as well to drug therapy).

Once Parkinson's develops, the problem is usually slowly progressive but its' course is variable. The rate varies in different patients but most patients will require levodopa therapy within two years of diagnosis. It should be noted that drug therapy is started earlier in patients who have other medical conditions such as arthritis, stroke and depression. Some patients and especially those with tremor of one arm may have a very mild form and require no treatment for a number of years. Overall, patients with tremor tend to have a milder type of Parkinson's.

Cause

The cause of Parkinson's is not fully understood. However for more than 30 years it has been known that its main symptoms are due to a deficiency in the production of a chemical called dopamine. This lack of **dopamine** is due to the death of dopamine producing cells in a region of the brain called the substantia nigra. **These neurons or cells connect and provide dopamine to the basal ganglia** (see diagram of the brain).

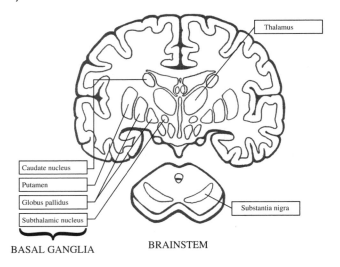

Thalamus

Caudate nucleus

Putamen

Globus pallidus

Subthalamic nucleus

BASAL GANGLIA

BRAINSTEM

Substantia nigra

Figure 1: The dopamine neurons that are affected in Parkinson's are in the substantia nigra of the brainstem. This area is connected to the basal ganglia and because of a loss of these cells, the caudate and putamen (also called the striatum) becomes deficient in dopamine. This results in parkinsonism.

The features of Parkinson's begin to be seen when 60 to 80% of the dopamine producing neurons are lost in the substantia nigra and there is an 80% reduction in dopamine in the basal ganglia. Unfortunately, it still is unclear why these specific cells die and many different potential factors are being actively investigated including: immune related factors; deficiencies of growth factors; accelerated aging processes; energy failure within the cells and "apoptosis" or programmed cell death. **These processes may be modified or initiated by genetic or environmental factors.**

Genetics

This is one of the most exciting areas of study in Parkinson's research at present. The recent identification of single gene defects in some forms of Parkinson's gives tremendous hope for the understanding of its cause. With the modern tools of molecular biology and molecular genetics, there have been major recent advances. **Genes control the production of proteins** and these proteins have many functions in normal cells. Some of these proteins are vital elements in the production of brain chemicals such as dopamine. If a gene is abnormal, then the proteins produced are not normal and vital cell functions may slow down leading eventually to cell death. It takes time to identify specific genes and their abnormalities. Once the gene is identified, it's function must be understood and then therapies must be developed and tested to either change or make up for the abnormal function.

Each step from gene identification to understanding and altering functions takes years but one can see the possibilities for prevention and treatment that will open up hopefully in the not too distant future. These strategies may include adding a gene that will increase or decrease the production of proteins with specific functions in cells.

There is increasing evidence that genetic factors play a role in the cause of Parkinson's. Apart from age, a positive family history of Parkinson's is the strongest predictor of an increased risk of developing the disease. A common way to try and sort out if there is a genetic component of a disease is to study twins. Identical twins share the same genes but non-identical twins share only half their genes (genes contain the information that makes up an individual characteristic including things like eye and hair color). If a disease has a strong genetic component then more sets of identical twins will have both twins affected versus the non-identical sets of twins. These types of studies have been done with sets of Parkinson's twins and do support the concept of a genetic component to the disease, especially for patients whose disease onsets before the age of 50.

For most families who have someone affected with Parkinson's, the increased risk of someone else developing it within the family is small when compared to the general population. However, there are a few rare families with multiple affected individuals that carry up to a 50% chance of someone within that family developing Parkinson's. In some of these rare families a specific genetic change has been identified that causes the disease within that family. A defect in a gene called "alpha-synuclein" was originally found in a large Italian and three Greek families. A different defect within the same gene was also found in one German family. To date, only eight families have been found that have alpha-synuclein gene defects and Parkinson's despite thousands of patients being screened for it. This suggests that defects in alpha-synuclein are an extremely rare cause for Parkinson's. **However it has**

produced important insights into the basic mechanisms of the disease. It has been found that the **Lewy body** (found in brain cells affected by Parkinson's) has a high concentration of alpha-synuclein and animal models of Parkinson's that have had gene manipulations to overproduce alpha-synuclein are being studied. It is felt that the mutation (gene defect) in alpha-synuclein leads to an **accumulation of protein, which forms the Lewy body** that disrupts the function of the dopamine producing neurons.

Two more abnormal genes named "parkin" and ubiquitin hydrolase have been associated with levodopa responsive parkinsonism. At this time it is unclear how changes in these genes result in the development of Parkinson's. Over the next few years more genes will almost surely be found.

It is as yet unknown how these newly identified genes in these rare families relate to most patients with Parkinson's but they will at the very least provide important clues **that will further our understanding of the mechanisms that are involved**. With our present knowledge for most families, the pattern of inheritance is not strong or clear enough that patients should be unduly worried about their children developing Parkinson's.

Summary of Parkinson's Genetics

The present status of our understanding is outlined below:

- Gene defects (along with other factors) play a role in the cause and predisposition to Parkinson's.

- Three abnormal genes have been identified and there are likely several more.

- Genes control the production of proteins that then control the function of cells (for example - dopamine production). Gene defects (along with other factors), play a role in the cause and predisposition to Parkinson's.

- If you are the only member of your family to have Parkinson's then it is very unlikely that you will pass it on to your children.

- Some rare families have multiple affected members and in these families the risk may be up to 50 percent. Even in these families if the gene is identified, not every person with the gene will develop Parkinson's. This makes counseling and prediction unclear and also sometimes the onset is delayed to very old age.

- At present there is no "blood test" for Parkinson's. The genetic tests are only done in research studies and there is just not enough known to give relatives any reliable results or advice from these tests alone.

Environmental Toxin Exposure

As everyone ages they slowly lose their dopamine producing cells and perhaps the development of Parkinson's is the **result of an event earlier in life** that killed a portion of these cells. Symptoms are then seen many years later when a **critical level of cell loss is reached as part of the normal aging process**. This event that occurred early in life may be an exposure to some environmental toxin. It is now known that specific toxins (e.g. MPTP) can precipitate Parkinson's but these toxins are rare and it is very unlikely that most people will have any exposure to them. MPTP when taken up by the body is converted into a toxic chemical called MPP+ and was originally found to cause Parkinson's disease in intravenous (IV) drug users. However, many more IV drug users were exposed to MPTP and did not develop Parkinson's suggesting **that other factors unique to certain individuals** also play a role even with this very toxic chemical. There have been many attempts to identify other toxins that are found more commonly in the environment that could increase your risk of developing Parkinson's but to date, **no specific ones have clearly been found**. Parkinson's has been shown to be more common in farmers and also in people who had occupational exposure to pesticides. Studies of possible gene defects in the system (in Parkinson's patients) that handles environmental toxins have proven negative. Interestingly, it has been noted that smoking protects against the development of Parkinson's. More recent detailed studies have shown no protective effects and also Parkinson's patients are more likely to quit smoking. The known harmful effects of smoking overshadow any possible protective effect. Overall, for most patients it is likely **that Parkinson's is the result of a combination of factors** that include genetic and environmental influences.

Young-Onset Parkinson's

Young-onset is defined as the onset of Parkinson's between the ages of 21 and 39. It involves about five percent of patients and seems to be basically the same illness as the older-onset type **but with the following differences**: progression of parkinsonian signs and symptoms is more gradual; dyskinesias and motor fluctuations tend to appear earlier; memory disturbances and mental side effects of medications seem to develop later; and dystonia (muscle spasm) is frequently present and is often a presenting sign. Independence and preservation of postural reflexes is often maintained for 20 or more years and young onset patients are frequently good candidates for surgery. Young onset Parkinson's seems to be **mainly restricted to the dopamine system** and therefore mobility is the main problem with a good response to medication.

The onset of Parkinson's in the teen years is termed juvenile onset and has much more dystonia and is much more in families. These are the patients where the "parkin" gene abnormality was originally found.

Management of Young-Onset Parkinson's

- Family and personal relationship stress is common and contributing factors include: financial concerns, depression, anxiety and sexual dysfunction. Psychological, financial and drug and medical benefit counseling may give very significant help and reassurance.

- Because of the greater tendency to have dystonia and early dyskinesias and motor fluctuations, strategies to delay levodopa use must be considered (see section on Current Drug Therapies). These include: amantadine, possibly anticholinergics (consider side effects) and dopamine agonists. When levodopa is needed, use the lowest dose that gives good symptom relief.

- Have an experienced Parkinson's neurologist directing your treatment.

Brain Scans

Special diagnostic tests are rarely helpful in confirming either the diagnosis of typical Parkinson's or of one of the atypical forms of parkinsonism. Parkinson's is **mainly a clinical diagnosis that is made by an experienced neurologist**. Special tests are undertaken if there are unusual symptoms or if the response to medication is poor. In these cases, the following diagnostic tests may be used in scanning the brain: computerized tomography (CT scan), magnetic resonance imaging (MRI scan), positron emission tomography (PET scan), and single photon emission computed tomography (SPECT scan).

Regular CT and MRI scans are normal in typical Parkinson's. Hydrocephalus (enlargement of the inner fluid filled cavities of the brain) or multiple small strokes can sometimes present with parkinsonian features and these changes can often be seen on either a CT or MRI scan. MRI is often helpful in atypical parkinsonism and in patients with unsatisfactory drug response. In some patients with multiple system atrophy (one type of atypical parkinsonism), the MRI may show: smallness of the brainstem (also seen in progressive supranuclear palsy); smallness of the cerebellum (the area of the brain that controls balance); small strokes; or possibly tissue density changes in the putamen (part of the basal ganglia). It can also show hydrocephalus and basal ganglia changes of Wilson's disease. In typical Parkinson's MR spectroscopy (shows cell function) is showing significant changes in the substantia nigra and basal ganglia and may eventually be useful in detecting the illness before symptoms develop.

PET and SPECT scans are at present **research tools**, which are being refined and will likely become more important. These tests use special markers which show specific dopamine functions if the brain. They are going to be helpful: in early diagnosis, making a more definite diagnosis and in following the results of treatment. These tests will be crucial in **testing neuroprotective therapies to slow or stop the progression of Parkinson's**. PET scanning is very expensive and not widely available, however most hospitals have equipment that can perform SPECT scans. These tests can show how much dopamine is being taken up, stored and released by certain parts of the brain. The **dopamine transporter** is the **best cell marker** for the basal ganglia dopamine cells most at risk in Parkinson's. SPECT can show a clear reduction of dopamine transporter in Parkinson's and this can be followed over time and will be able to measure progression or slowing of progression with new therapies. All of these brain-scanning advances will assist in developing and assessing new therapies for patients with Parkinson's.

Types of Parkinsonism and Disorders Which May Be Confused With Parkinson's

The term "parkinsonism" refers to a group of disorders in which patients notice tremor, slow movements, stiffness of the limbs and difficulty walking. The **most common slowly progressive condition that causes parkinsonism is Parkinson's disease itself**. However, essential tremor is often misdiagnosed as Parkinson's disease and a drug induced form of parkinsonism is also very common. There is a large group of conditions that make up the atypical or pseudo parkinsonism group. **In this**

book we will refer to Parkinson's disease as Parkinson's. It is also called classic Parkinson's or idiopathic (cause not known) or primary or Lewy body Parkinson's (the Lewy body is seen in the abnormal dopamine neurons). Parkinson's and its main mimickers (other types of parkinsonism) are described below.

Classical Parkinson's disease

The most typical form of parkinsonism is made up of **four main** symptoms and signs: resting tremor, rigidity, bradykinesia and loss of balance (postural instability). The patient's **earliest complaints may include** fatigue, general slowness, small handwriting, poor hand co-ordination, and a tremulous feeling in one arm with or without observable tremor. **The best markers that a patient may have Parkinson's are**: symptoms begin on one side, rest tremor is present and the patient responds well to levodopa therapy.

Essential Tremor

While features of parkinsonism (stiffness and slowness) are lacking in this disorder, the tremor that it causes is sometimes confused with parkinsonian tremor. The major difference though is that the tremor of Parkinson's occurs at rest and stops or becomes less noticeable when active movement is attempted. **Essential tremor, on the other hand, occurs when the hands are held in a particular posture, such as holding a cup (postural tremor) or when the limb is moved towards an object (action tremor)**. Essential tremor is much more common than Parkinson's and can occur at any age. It is estimated that up to 20 percent of people over age 70 may have mild essential tremor.

The following features can distinguish it:

- The tremor occurs with posture and action (when the hand is being used or held in a particular posture)
- Head tremor is common and voice tremor may occur
- Rigidity, bradykinesia and gait disorder are absent
- There is often a family history of essential tremor
- The patient usually has a longer history of tremor
- The tremor may improve dramatically with small amounts of alcohol

Patients with a family history of essential tremor usually only have hand action tremor and not dystonia (a more sustained abnormal contraction of muscles), or head or voice tremor. Some older patients with longstanding essential tremor have a slight rest tremor and some tone increase; but the absence of bradykinesia will rule out significant Parkinson's. **Some patients with classic Parkinson's will also have postural and action tremor**. Therefore, some patients may have both conditions together so that it may not always be easy to distinguish between these disorders. Recent studies have raised the question of whether there is a link between essential tremor and Parkinson's. There is no consensus on this at present. Treatment with levodopa is not effective for essential tremor but it can be aided with two medications: propranolol or primidone. Both of these drugs should be introduced cautiously (see section on Drug Therapies). Patients with essential tremor frequently (50%) have some impairment of tandem walking (walking with one foot in front of the other).

Drug Induced Parkinsonism

Drugs that block dopamine receptors are capable of inducing a parkinsonian-like illness. The most common culprits in the past have been drugs (neuroleptics) used to treat serious mental illness. **Drug induced parkinsonism however is now seen with a great number of newer medications**. It is seen more in older individuals and it has been suggested that those who develop it may have pre-existing brain dopamine deficiency and these patients have been shown to have various abnormalities in the substantia nigra that increase their risk of drug induced parkinsonism. **It usually develops in the first few months of drug use**, it is worse on one side and involves the upper body more. Significant disability may develop quite quickly in drug induced parkinsonism as opposed to the slow progression of true Parkinson's. The severity increases with longer time on the drug.

Some **drugs used for stomach disorders**; metoclopramide has been a frequent culprit; also clebopride (available in Europe) have caused parkinsonism. Drugs used for hallucinations and agitation can cause parkinsonism or aggravate existing Parkinson's (see drugs discussed in section on Confusion and Hallucinations).

Calcium channel blockers that are widely used for a number of illnesses (heart disease, high blood pressure) have the ability to interfere with dopamine transmission at multiple stages. Drugs of this class include: diltiazem; nifedipine; verapamil; manipidine; captopril; amlodipine; and flunarizine (cinnarizine) which has been widely used in Mexico, Spain and South America. All of these drugs can cause parkinsonism and some also cause muscle jerking (myoclonus) and foot and toe cramping (dystonia). Considering the widespread use of these drugs for cardiovascular illness and their benefits, the Parkinson's patient on a calcium channel blocker must be carefully evaluated. The risk of inducing or aggravating parkinsonism is real, but small.

Selective serotonin reuptake inhibitors are drugs that increase serotonin in the brain and treat depression and are commonly used in Parkinson's. These drugs may cause or aggravate parkinsonism in a small number of patients. It may be that other factors are involved such as also being on selegiline. Drugs of this type include: sertraline, paroxetine, fluvoxamime and fluoxetine (Prozac). Prozac should not be used, as it has been a much more frequent culprit. The others are helpful medications for depressed Parkinson's patients but the low risk or motor worsening should be watched for after they are started.

Meperidine (Demerol) may cause acute parkinsonism that may require short term levodopa to clear. This has occurred in non-Parkinson's patients and the drug should not be used in patients with Parkinson's.

The chronic use of valproate (Depakene) may cause a reversible combination of parkinsonism and cognitive impairment that may take up to 12 months to develop. It increases in severity with age and may be associated with hearing loss.

Amiodarone, a potent drug to treat abnormal cardiac rhythms has caused parkinsonism. Other drugs implicated include:

vincristine and cytosine arabinoside (anti-cancer drugs); Dilantin; lithium; and alpha-methyldopa. Alcohol withdrawal may cause parkinsonism. The hallucinogen "ecstasy" has been the suspected cause in at least one patient.

Improvement of drug-induced parkinsonism can take weeks to months after the withdrawal of the drug and after long term use there is a risk of unpleasant involuntary face and body movements (tardive dyskinesias). **In any patient with parkinsonism, all drugs should be carefully reviewed and drug induced parkinsonism must be considered and excluded**.

Atypical Parkinsonism or Parkinson's Plus

It is important to distinguish between Parkinson's and its imitators. Illnesses that resemble Parkinson's are individually rare but collectively these look-alikes may account for **up to 20% of patients with parkinsonism**. Often the diagnosis is difficult in the first few years of the illness. These patients have parkinsonian symptoms resulting from a number of disorders, most of unknown cause. It is important to try and define the look-alikes. Patients can be given a more definite diagnosis and outlook for the future. The treatment is often different, correct drug use may avoid unnecessary drug costs and side effects and proper classification will aid research and eventually trials of therapies to prevent progression. If a patient has parkinsonian features with additional disabilities not seen regularly or as severe in classical Parkinson's, then it may indicate that another illness is occurring.

These atypical disorders tend to cause earlier and more severe disability. The presence of some of the following features may help to differentiate these atypical forms of parkinsonism from classical Parkinson's:

- Early onset and greater predominance of unsteady gait, postural defects and falls

- Rapid progression

- Absence of typical parkinsonian resting tremor

- Early onset of memory problems

- Atypical or severe rigidity with dystonic features (twisting involuntary movements)

- Neck flexion' chin on chest

- Early onset of dizziness associated with low blood pressure (postural hypotension is a drop in blood pressure on standing)

- Early onset of bladder dysfunction (often called neurogenic bladder) and sexual dysfunction in both males and females

- Abnormal foot (plantar) responses and deep tendon reflexes

- Impaired eye (extraocular) movements or eye opening

- Poor or waning response to levodopa therapy and absence of typical drug induced dyskinesias

Because of the multiple problems that develop, patients with these atypical disorders need careful assessment and follow-up care. There are many things that can be done to improve comfort, mobility and quality of life.

There are a number of conditions that may produce atypical parkinsonism. These are outlined below.

Progressive Supranuclear Palsy

This condition typically begins with **gait problems** and **spontaneous backward falls** often in the first year of symptoms. It is more common in men. When examined, patients will often be unable to look down (although they may not be aware of this) and this causes problems walking down stairs. **Other eye problems include**: double vision; blurred vision; difficulty reading; burning eyes; light sensitivity; slowing of eye opening and closing; and inability to open the eyes at will. Difficulty with speech and swallowing are common early in this disorder as is the tendency for the eyes to close spontaneously (blepharospasm). Significant rest tremor is usually absent. Depression, slowed thinking, word finding difficulty and reduced concentration occur in some but not all patients. There is often a history of high blood pressure and sleep upset with frequent wakenings may be present. This disorder is progressive and unfortunately, the response to drugs is not as good as in typical Parkinson's. Blepharospasm may respond well to local injections into the eyelid muscles (with botulism toxin).

Multiple System Atrophy

This is the most common cause of mistaken diagnosis of Parkinson's. The initial symptoms are: slowness, unsteadiness, walking difficulty, bladder and sexual dysfunction and light-headedness. Only about 5% of patients have early tremor and over time only 15% have rest tremor (45% have various non-typical tremors). Other problems that develop are: low volume voice, excess saliva, swallowing difficulty, poor handwriting, and bowel and respiratory dysfunction. **Blood pressure often becomes a major problem** with drops on standing that may cause unconsciousness. Antiparkinson drugs aggravate this and often the blood pressure varies (increases lying down) and patients are placed on antihypertensive medication, which further lowers the standing blood pressure. These patients should always have their pressure checked lying and standing. There is often some response to levodopa but the patient is frequently more disabled by poor balance than by slowness. Some patients have no motor response to levodopa yet develop dyskinesias.

Multiple system atrophy in the past was separated into three supposedly distinct conditions but it was increasingly recognized there was frequently overlap between them. If patients had more stiffness and no tremor the term **striatonigral degeneration** was used. If prominent early unsteadiness was one of the main features the term **olivopontocerebellar degeneration** was used and if in addition the patient had prominent early sexual dysfunction and blood pressure drops on standing the term **Shy-drager syndrome** was used.

Corticobasal degeneration (CBD)

This is an uncommon disorder, which shows marked stiffness, complex sensory defects and jerky movements. Treatment is difficult with modest response to levodopa and myoclonus (muscle jerks) may benefit from clonazepam.

Vascular Parkinsonism

This involves the **legs more than arms** and presents with stiff, slow, short step walking (lower body parkinsonism) and the onset may be fairly acute. **Freezing is common**. It is caused by multiple small strokes and is seen in patients with high blood pressure and vascular disease. Usually there is no tremor and the response to levodopa is variable but it should always be tried as some patients have an excellent response (especially with substantia nigra stroke). Some patients with typical Parkinson's may have clearing of one-sided tremor, stiffness and dyskinesias with a small stroke on the opposite side of the brain.

Post Traumatic Parkinsonism

This is seen in boxers and is related to the number of bouts not knockouts. In addition to variable signs of parkinsonism these patients have memory and behavioural upsets. It may onset decades after the last fight and is rarely seen after single head injuries. Blows cause damage to the substantia nigra. The response to medication is less predictable than typical Parkinson's.

Wilson's Disease

This is a rare genetically determined defect in copper metabolism **that must be tested for as it is treatable**. Copper deposits occur in the liver, brain and cornea. The disease is seen in younger patients almost always under age 50. A low blood level of a copper transport protein (ceruloplasmin) and increased copper in a 24-hour urine collection diagnose it. A MRI scan will often show density changes in the basal ganglia.

The gene defect for Wilson's Disease (involved in copper transport) has been identified and can help confirm the diagnosis if the basic tests are positive. A liver biopsy is sometimes necessary. **Every patient under age 50 with symptoms of parkinsonism should be tested.**

Parkinsonism with Prominent Memory Difficulties

See section on Memory Disorders

Parkinsonism with Hydrocephalus

This is rare and is diagnosed by a CT scan. The patient has prominent memory loss usually without tremor. Management is complex, the surgery to try and reduce the abnormally large fluid filled cavities within the brain is not always successful. Some patients eventually develop typical Parkinson's which is difficult to manage because of the memory and thinking impairment.

Very Early Symptoms of Parkinson's

Some patients experience very early symptoms of Parkinson's, that may occur four to six years before classic Parkinson's is diagnosed. **Some of these early symptoms may include**: depression; scattered pains (especially in the shoulder and low back), cramps and numbness; constipation or diarrhea; hypertension; internal tremor (see section on Pain and Sensory Symptoms) and decreased sense of smell. The scattered pains, cramps and numbness usually improve after the initiation of levodopa.

Tests are being developed to **try and diagnose very early classical Parkinson's** so that new treatments that delay or stop progression of the disease can be tried and evaluated.

There are an increasing number of medications that can treat the symptoms of Parkinson's, but unfortunately **none that are currently available clearly slow the progression of the disease**. Whether selegiline (Deprenyl), a monoamine oxidase-B (MAO-B) enzyme inhibitor, really slows the progression of Parkinson's, as originally claimed, or simply reduces the symptoms of the disease remains controversial but the large studies show that it does not slow progression. In the early stage of Parkinson's when symptoms are noticed but not troublesome, symptomatic treatment is not necessary, remembering that all drugs have the potential to induce side effects. In general, **it is appropriate to start treatment** when a patient begins to experience functional difficulties that result in a reduced quality of life, impairment in the performance of activities of daily living or are a threat to employment status (usually by about year two). This decision needs to be individualized as each patient has different views of what constitutes sufficient functional impairment to impact on quality of life. However, it must be remembered that delaying effective symptomatic therapy beyond a point of significant disability has been shown to result in an increased mortality.

Once the decision has been made to initiate treatment **one could consider starting with a less potent** (and effective) agent including selegiline, amantadine or one of the anticholinergics (used infrequently now). When greater symptomatic benefit is required, **it is well accepted that levodopa** (usually taken in the form of Sinemet or Prolopa) is the most effective method of reducing parkinsonian disability. The number of available drugs has made treatment more complex and their use must be tailored to each patient individually. Younger patients because they are more likely to have motor complications will benefit **from delaying the use of levodopa and should be treated early with a dopamine agonist** when more potent therapy is needed. Patients must remember that all drugs have side effects and antiparkinsonian drugs are no exception. To minimize these side effects patients must start slowly with these drugs, working up gradually from low doses. **Smaller doses and more caution for adverse effects should be the drug rules for older patients**. If a drug does not seem to be effective, then it should be withdrawn before another is started. Drugs interact with each other; the more drugs you are on the more side effects are likely. However, most patients with moderate parkinsonian disability require several drugs to control their symptoms.

Where possible we have used the generic name of the drug rather than the brand (company) name. However, some drugs are better known by their brand name such as Sinemet (levodopa) and we often interchange them. Others are known by their generic name, for example bromocriptine.

Note: Manipulations of the following drugs should not be undertaken by the patient alone but in consultation with your doctor. You should feel free to suggest changes to your doctor or neurologist. Patients should have a neurologist participating in their care and if possible should have regular assessments by a Parkinson's-movement disorder specialist and clinic.

Levodopa and its Complications

Levodopa is converted to dopamine in the brain. **Dopamine is the deficient chemical in Parkinson's** but it cannot be used directly, as it cannot easily cross into the brain. Levodopa (L-dopa) helps reduce rigidity and tremor, and is most effective in combating **bradykinesia** (slowness of movement). Levodopa is the mainstay of treatment and is the best drug available. Almost all patients can take levodopa and almost all parkinsonian patients will eventually be treated with it.

Is levodopa toxic?

There has been growing concern raised in both the medical and the lay press that levodopa may be toxic to dopamine cells. The evidence for this is mainly derived from experiments where dopamine cells are grown in the laboratory in isolation and levodopa is placed with the cells. In these experiments, the dopamine cells exposed to high concentrations of levodopa die faster than the cells not exposed to levodopa suggesting a toxic effect of levodopa. However, if the same experiments are performed with the addition of the normal supporting cells found in the brain this toxic effect is not seen and the predominant effect may in fact be protective. **Studies in healthy animals have consistently failed to demonstrate that levodopa is toxic** and it has been shown to actually prolong the life span of some mice.

There are **no studies in humans** that demonstrate that long-term administration of levodopa damages dopamine cells. Non-parkinsonian patients exposed to levodopa for many years have not shown damage to their dopamine cells at autopsy.

Human studies have shown that the administration of levodopa has improved the life expectancy of patients with Parkinson's and may slow disease progression. With time, some patients develop symptoms that are poorly responsive to levodopa therapy such as speech, memory and thinking difficulties, problems with walking and balance difficulties. Whether levodopa contributes to the development of these symptoms is unknown but it is more likely they are secondary to disease-related loss of additional cells outside the dopamine system.

Even though levodopa is **not truly toxic** to **dopamine cells, patients taking it do develop a variety of complications that become a major therapeutic challenge over time** (see next section). The cause of these levodopa-related motor complications is poorly understood and concerns regarding these problems have contributed to the longstanding debate on whether or not levodopa treatment should be delayed. Individuals treated (having a wrong diagnosis) with levodopa that have a normal dopamine system (e.g. essential tremor) do not develop these levodopa-related motor complications even after prolonged exposure. Parkinson's patients did not have these types of motor fluctuations prior to the discovery of levodopa but they were recognized soon after levodopa was introduced. The current dose of levodopa clearly plays a role in the severity of levodopa induced abnormal movements (dyskinesias) since they improve or resolve on lowering the dose.

The **duration of levodopa treatment also contributes to these motor complications** as demonstrated in one study where the complications increased from 20% in the first five years to 70% after 15 years of treatment. Age of onset of the disease also has an effect on the occurrence of these problems. Patients with young-onset Parkinson's (under the age of 40) have an increased risk of developing dyskinesias and motor fluctuations and this has encouraged many neurologists to delay the introduction of levodopa as long as possible in this group. Overall, it seems likely that the **motor complications seen with long term levodopa therapy are in part the result of levodopa therapy and also are related to progression of the disease with increasing loss of dopamine neurons.**

In Conclusion:

- Levodopa is the most effective treatment for parkinsonian symptoms and it decreases mortality rate and may slow progression

- There is no evidence that the long term use of levodopa worsens the brain process of Parkinson's

- Levodopa induced fluctuations and dyskinesias result from both brain dopamine neuron malfunction (for which there is no treatment at present) and the dose and use of levodopa (which can be adjusted)

- In summary there is no cause for concern that levodopa is dangerous for patients.

Levodopa is commonly used **in combination** with either carbidopa (Sinemet) or benserazide (Prolopa) because of their help in stopping levodopa from changing to dopamine before reaching the brain. These combination preparations are more effective and allow about 80 percent less levodopa to be used. This helps reduce nausea, low blood pressure on standing (postural hypotension) and heart problems as was seen in patients who took plain levodopa. In these combination preparations, the lower number indicates the amount (mg) of carbidopa, and the larger number represents the amount of levodopa. i.e. Sinemet 100/25 tablet contains 100 mg of levodopa and 25 mg of carbidopa (in the United States the numbers are in reverse order). Controlled-release Sinemet (Sinemet CR) is a levodopa preparation that is very helpful for the fluctuating symptoms of Parkinson's. Sinemet CR is a combination of levodopa and carbidopa which slowly dissolves in the stomach and gives a reduction in motor fluctuations (see section on Daily Mobility Fluctuations). Greater periods of mobility ("on" time), and a more predictable day have been noted. It is a very useful drug for end of dose failure ("wearing off" effect), as the total number of doses taken per day can often be reduced. The main problem with Sinemet CR has been the slower **onset of action compared to regular Sinemet**. The overall daily dose of levodopa is increased by about 30% when Sinemet CR is used because of its incomplete absorption. Injectable and new oral forms of levodopa (levodopa ethylester) are currently being studied in patients with severe response fluctuations (see section on Research and New Therapies).

Levodopa should be started slowly, taken after food and slowly increased to an initial low dose to await benefit. A common pattern is to start with Sinemet 100/25; take 1/2 tablet 1-3 times daily and add 1/2 tablet every 5-7 days until a total dose of 2-3 full tablets daily is achieved (see medication tips and schedules). Initial mild nausea usually clears quickly. If more severe gastric upset is not helped with small doses after food, then the drug domperidone (see section on Drug Related Nausea and Vomiting) should be used. Changing from Sinemet to Prolopa and vice versa occasionally helps this, and the rare occurrence of diarrhea, on levodopa initiation.

Less fatigue, improved general well being, faster movements and better walking are usually the first benefits. Tremor improves less. The dose should be adjusted upwards slowly depending on the patient's response. The initial use of large tablet sizes (Sinemet 250/25) and high doses is not recommended. Levodopa rarely causes confusion initially, but if it occurs, the drug should be reduced or temporarily stopped and all drugs reviewed.

Common Drug Name	Generic Drug Name	Daily Dosage (Milligrams)
Sinemet	Levodopa/Carbidopa	200 - 2500
Prolopa (Madopar)	levodopa/benserazide	250 - 2000
Larodopa	levodopa	3000-8000
Atamet (generic Sinemet)	levodopa/carbidopa	200-2500

Sinemet is available in five preparations (tablets)
100/10 mg (levodopa/carbidopa)
100/25 mg (most commonly used)
250/25 mg
CR 200/50 mg (CR = controlled or slow release)
CR 100/25 mg (CR= controlled or slow release)

Prolopa is available in four preparations (capsules):

50/12.5 mg (levodopa/benserazide)
100/25 mg
200/50 mg
Madopar HBS (HBS = slow release)

Main Early Side Effects

• nausea and vomiting (less than 10 percent)

• anorexia (loss of appetite for food)

• disturbed sleep/upsetting dreams

• dyskinesias (rare initially)

Note: Sinemet CR should not be chewed or crushed. This disturbs the ability to release the drug slowly. The tablet may be broken in half on a physician's instructions.

Example of a Schedule for Starting Levodopa Therapy

Continue all other medication as instructed by your doctor.

Sinemet   100/25 mg.

Take 1/2 tablet with food three times a day.

Add 1/2 tablet every 7 days until you are taking 1 tablet(s) three times a day.

Week Number	Breakfast	Lunch	Dinner
1	1/2	1/2	1/2
2	1	1/2	1/2
3	1	1	1/2
4	1	1	1

Long-term levodopa therapy is associated with certain problems but there is no evidence that early or prolonged use of levodopa advances the progression of Parkinson's; it is clear that it enhances survival.

Outlined below are problems that can develop during levodopa use:

Daily Mobility Fluctuations

Initially the improvement with levodopa seems even and stable over a day. After months or years of treatment, patients begin to note a **return of parkinsonism three to five hours after their last dose**. This is more common and severe in younger patients. Levodopa absorption varies considerably throughout the day. It seems that absorption becomes less consistent in the afternoon and evening, which could lead to a worsening of parkinsonian symptoms (see section on Impaired Gastric Emptying). In addition there are changes in the storage and handling of dopamine in the brain because of the loss of dopamine nerve terminals and the handling of levodopa in the rest of the body is also altered. **There are several types of mobility fluctuations including:**

End-Of-Dose Failure ("wearing off" effect)

This means a return of parkinsonian symptoms before the next dose of levodopa is due. It may not occur after each dose, is more common later in the day and may be delayed for five to six hours in the first few years of treatment. The "wearing off" effect is **most likely related to the state of dopamine producing cells in the brain when treatment is started**. If there is more loss of cells and a lower level of dopamine, then end-of-dose failure may be more prominent.

This loss of effect may vary from patient to patient. For some, there is a subtle increase in slowness or tremor, and for others there is a complete inability to walk. The wearing-off effect may vary in duration from a few minutes to hours. Relief of these disabilities usually comes only with the next dose of levodopa and there is often a delay of 30 to 60 minutes until the next dose is absorbed from the stomach and reaches the brain.

"On-Off" Phenomenon

This is a rapid, unpredictable, appearance and disappearance of the beneficial side effects of levodopa therapy. **The patient fluctuates from mobility to sudden immobility**. "On" is used to describe the condition when a person is responding optimally to his or her medications. During "on" periods, a person can move about and perform activities of daily living with relative ease. The mobile phase ("on") is commonly accompanied with, or disturbed by dyskinesias. "Off" is used to describe the period of time when a patient is having more difficulty with movement. **The "on-off" phenomenon is the most severe type of fluctuation and only affects about 10%**

of patients with fluctuations. The "off" phase usually lasts for ten to fifteen minutes or longer. This fluctuation is unpredictable and not clearly related to levodopa dose timing. It is more difficult to treat than wearing off but most of the same medication adjustments should be tried. Slow release levodopa preparation should be avoided in the unpredictable "off" patients.

Freezing

Patients with Parkinson's may develop sudden brief (seconds) periods of immobility called freezing. This problem is felt to be more a part of the illness and related to progression rather than a levodopa complication. These periods may occur when movement is initiated or altered and can be categorised into four types:

- Sudden transient freezing in the middle of walking

- Start-hesitation such as rising from a chair and then being unable to step forward

- Turning-hesitation when trying to change direction

- Terminal-hesitation when the patient is unable to complete a final action such as sitting down or stepping up onto a weight scale.

Many of these freezing periods occur when the patient is suddenly distracted or interrupted during an ongoing movement (see sections on Gait and Tips to Initiate Movement). The problem may occur during levodopa "wearing off spells" in which case it responds to increased medication. It may also occur during "on times" and it is **important to decide** if the patient is **underdosed** (and needs more medication) **or overdosed** and an overall reduction in medication is needed. It is seen more in patients without tremor and with lower body parkinsonism.

No "On" Response

In advanced disease, fluctuating patients may occasionally fail to respond to a given dose of levodopa. This is known as the no "on" response and is usually due to inadequate absorption of levodopa. This can be caused by an inadequate dose, slowing of GI (gastrointestinal) transit time, and competition for levodopa absorption from dietary protein (see section on Impaired Gastric Emptying).

Less Common Fluctuations

There are several other, less familiar types of fluctuating changes which Parkinson patients may experience. Many of these symptoms **are non-motor in nature but are usually associated with motor fluctuations** (slow spells). These other fluctuations include:

- Pain and numbness in the legs or arms. Abdominal pain may also occur

- Restless legs

- Sweating

- Urinary frequency

- Drooling and increased difficulty swallowing

- Depression, anxiety, reduced memory and hallucinations. Some patients have also experienced panic, hyperventilation, moaning and screaming while in an "off" period

- Shortness of breath

- Yawning - just before an "on" spell

One patient may have a number of the above symptoms and it is important that family and caregivers recognize them. Treatment to reduce motor fluctuations may improve these symptoms.

It has been noted that some women may have up to a 50% worsening of motor fluctuations for a few days before and during menstrual periods. This has been remarkably improved with Diamox (acetazolamide) 500 mg. daily taken 2 to 3 days before and during menstruation (total of 6 to 8 days).

These various daily mobility fluctuations may be managed by your doctor with the following strategies:

- Add a dopamine agonist using low initial doses, decrease levodopa early if dyskinesias increase, and be prepared to give 3-4 doses of dopamine agonist with levodopa 4-6 times daily

- Use a slow release levodopa preparation (Sinemet CR)

- Supplement Sinemet CR with regular Sinemet

- Add a COMT inhibitor

- Use more frequent, smaller doses of levodopa (often without increased daily dosage)

- Chew or break the tablets of regular Sinemet (100-25) which can help speed up the onset of effect

- Chew the tablets of regular Sinemet (100-25) and take them with a carbonated beverage which may further speed the onset of action

- Try liquid levodopa (see below)

- Observe the impact of high protein meals on the levodopa effect (see section on Weight Loss, Nutrition and the Low Protein Diet)

- Consider surgical procedure

- See section on Tips to Initiate Movement

Other methods to enhance the effectiveness of levodopa include:

- Inserting a tube through the wall of the abdomen and directly into the small bowel for direct delivery of levodopa. This will also help nutrition if swallowing is poor. It should be done very infrequently.

- Preparing levodopa in a liquid form and drinking it on a 1 or 2 hour basis (this is only done under careful supervision and most patients find it very cumbersome).

- Enhancing gastric motility with drugs, such as cisapride (see section on Impaired Gastric Emptying for the last two methods).

Involuntary Movements (Dyskinesias)

Dyskinesias are **involuntary movements** of the face, arms, legs, or trunk and should not be confused with tremor. Tremor is more smooth and rhythmic whereas dyskinesias tend to be jerky (chorea) and twisting (dystonia). Dyskinesias are often more prominent in more advanced patients and are worse on the more affected side. Family may first observe these movements as restlessness (especially in the legs) or an inability to sit still.

Involuntary movements caused by levodopa treatment occur in up to 80% of patients with longstanding Parkinson's. These movements frequently occur with mobility fluctuations such as "wearing off" and "on-off" effects. It has been found that dyskinesias are worsened with stress or activity.

The basic principle is that pulses of levodopa stimulation acting on sensitized dopamine receptors cause involuntary movements. **If the dose is reduced, they will decrease, but parkinsonism may be worse. Dopamine agonists cause less dyskinesias than levodopa and the probability of developing dyskinesias is less in patients who are only on dopamine agonist therapy and this is why they are preferred for early treatment**. It has now been shown that the early use of antioxidants such as Vitamin E or the early use of selegiline **does not protect** against the onset of dyskinesias and motor fluctuations.

There are several patterns of dyskinesias including:

Peak-Dose Dyskinesias

This is the earliest and most common form dyskinesias and occurs at the peak of levodopa's effect. **Patients tend to have the maximum involuntary movements when they are most active**. In the early stages the dyskinesias are usually well tolerated and are easy to control by reducing the individual doses of levodopa. However, as the disease advances patients do not tolerate this reduction in levodopa and other strategies must be tried (see below).

Diphasic dyskinesias (or Onset and End of Dose Dyskinesias)

Ten to fifteen percent of patients develop diphasic dyskinesias. Diphasic dyskinesias are those which occur shortly after taking levodopa when the antiparkinsonian effect commences, and also occur when the effect of the drug is wearing off. Beginning dyskinesias are followed by an "on" period, while end-of-dose dyskinesias are followed by an "off" period. The pattern of diphasic dyskinesia is often characterized as: **dyskinesia** (going on) - **improvement** (on) - **dyskinesia** (going off) but some patients only have the "going on" or "going off" phase. Severe leg kicking is a common pattern. The use of Sinemet CR for this type of dyskinesia is not recommended, as it will prolong the duration of the dyskinesias and sometimes make them almost continuous.

Dystonia

Dystonia is another type of involuntary movement where **more continuous muscular contractions** occur. Dystonia may be diphasic, peak, or end of dose. It is more sustained when levodopa effect wears off (off-period dystonia) and more intermittent and brief at the peak of effect. Dystonia can occur before patients are treated with levodopa, but is usually treatment related. It usually involves the head and neck, with head turning, facial contraction, eyelid blinking or tongue thrusting outwards.

Early morning and off-period dystonia, usually occurring in the feet or legs, is characterized by painful muscle contractions, similar to cramps. It is related to low levodopa levels and is worse on the side most affected by parkinsonism.

When early morning foot dystonic movements occur, your doctor can try the following:

• A slow release preparation of levodopa taken the night before

• A dopamine agonist taken the night before

• A dose of levodopa on wakening (chew for faster absorption)

• Lithium

• Botulinum toxin injections

When "peak dose" dystonic movements occur, the following can be tried:

• Lower the dose of levodopa

• Add or increase a dopamine agonist with a decrease in levodopa

• Botulinum toxin injections

• Consider surgical procedure

When "wearing off or off period" dystonic movements occur, see section below on treatment suggestions for daily mobility fluctuations.

Akathisia (Restlessness)

Akathisia occurs in one quarter of Parkinson's patients and in patients with fluctuations and it can appear in the on or off phases but most commonly in the wearing off period. It is seen as **restlessness or an inability to sit or lie still** and is associated with an urge to move. This is different from dyskinesias, when patients may not be aware of their movements. It can occur before levodopa treatment begins but usually occurs after treatment. It may be a serious problem at night, causing insomnia. Minor tranquilizers (clonazepam) and dopamine agonists have given benefit if levodopa adjustments fail. Restless leg syndrome (see section on Sleep) is much more bothersome.

When dyskinesias occur, your doctor may try the following:

- Reduce levodopa or use more frequent smaller doses of levodopa

- Add amantadine

- Combine a dopamine agonist with a reduced dose of levodopa

- Reduce or stop selegiline

- Reduce or stop anticholinergics and observe the possible effect of other drugs with anticholinergic effects like antidepressants and bladder drugs (Ditropan is an unlikely factor)

- Consider liquid levodopa

- Clozapine

- Consider a surgical procedure

The newest drug treatment concept to reduce dyskinesias is to inhibit NMDA receptors (see section on Amantadine) with amantadine and also dextromethorphan (used cautiously in recent experimental studies). All these drug manipulations should be tried before consideration of surgery and newer drugs are being tested.

Dopamine Agonists

Dopamine agonists are a class of medications that are not converted to dopamine in the brain (as levodopa is), but instead bind directly to the receptors of cells to improve the symptoms of Parkinson's (see figure 2). In other words, **dopamine agonists mimic some of the effects of dopamine in the brain by directly stimulating dopamine receptors**. We now know that there are at least five subtypes of dopamine receptors. This can be understood by imagining that dopamine fits like a key into five different locks (receptors) on the walls of brain cells. Drugs are being developed that selectively block, or turn on, just one or two locks.

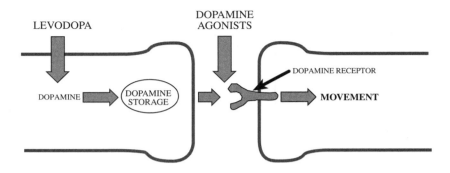

Figure 2: A schematic comparison of how levodopa and dopamine agonists work. On the left is the nerve cell that normally produces the dopamine and is lost in Parkinson's patients (the cells of the substantia nigra). On the right is the cell that normally receives the dopamine (the cells of the caudate and putamen).

There are currently **four** different oral dopamine agonists available for the treatment of Parkinson's disease. The "old" dopamine agonists include **bromocriptine** (Parlodel) and **pergolide** (Permax) and the two "new" dopamine agonists that have just become available: **ropinirole** (Requip) and **pramipexole** (Mirapex). Cabergoline, another new, very long acting dopamine agonist, has been shown to be effective but currently is not being marketed for Parkinson's disease in North America. **They have all been shown to be effective and are preferred in the early stages of Parkinson's, as the incidence of dyskinesias and fluctuations is less compared to levodopa**. The majority of patients will however eventually require the addition of levodopa. In later stages they can improve motor fluctuations and reduce off-times and have less of a tendency to cause dyskinesias than levodopa. The newer dopamine agonists are also being investigated to see if they can slow the progression of the disease. There are very few studies that have compared dopamine agonists against each other but there is a suggestion that the new ones may be more potent than bromocriptine in their ability to improve symptoms. It has been shown that it is safe and easier to switch quickly (rather than slowly over weeks) from an older agonist to one of the new ones. The plan is: calculate equivalent dose; stop one day; start the new dopamine agonist the next day; and make further adjustments.

Dopamine agonists are more expensive than levodopa, are less potent especially in later stages of the disease, are more complex to use, usually take longer to reach effective doses and have more side effects. **However, because they cause less dyskinesias and motor fluctuations they are increasingly being used alone in the early stages of the disease especially in younger patients**. **The most frequent adverse side effects** are nausea and vomiting, light-headedness on standing (postural hypotension), drowsiness, constipation and psychiatric reactions (hallucinations and confusion). The nausea and postural hypotension tend to occur with the initiation of treatment and reduce as tolerance develops over days to weeks. The psychiatric adverse events require that caution be used in prescribing dopamine agonists in older patients or in patients with pre-existing psychiatric symptoms. Serious but infrequent adverse events associated with the older dopamine agonists (bromocriptine, pergolide are ergot derivatives) include lung and abdominal wall thickening (fibrosis) and erythromelalgia, (a painful reddish skin discoloration over the legs), and some caution in patients with blood vessel disease, are unlikely with the newer dopamine agonists (pramipexole and ropinirole).

Daytime sleepiness has occurred with pramipexole and ropinirole in a minority of patients. However sudden irresistible attacks of sleep have been reported with these drugs (more with pramipexole) and have resulted in car accidents. Patients who drive should be warned. Most of these patients did not have daytime sleepiness.

Dopamine agonists are complicated to use and therapy should be started under the supervision of an experienced neurologist. The basic principles of their use are: start at a very low dosage, slowly increase and often reduce levodopa at the same time. It is important to understand that the agonists rarely provide symptom relief at the lowest dose levels and one should not become discouraged or discontinue therapy. It may require several weeks of gradually increasing the dose before benefits are seen. These medications should not be stopped suddenly as this can cause a significant deterioration in symptoms and can result in a life threatening medical emergency (called the neuroleptic malignant-like syndrome). Symptoms of this include: a fever, confusion and a marked increase in stiffness throughout the body.

Common Drug Name	Generic Drug Name	Daily Dosage (Milligrams)
Parlodel	bromocriptine 2.5 mg tablets 5.0 mg capsules	5 - 60
Permax	pergolide 0.05mg tablets 0.25mg tablets 1.0mg tablets	0.1 - 5
Requip	ropinirole 0.25 mg tablets 0.5 mg tablets* 1 mg tablets 2 mg tablets 5 mg tablets	3 - 24
Mirapex	pramipexole 0.125 mg tablets* 0.25 mg tablets 0.5 mg tablets* 1.0 mg tablets 1.5 mg tablets	1.5 - 4.5

* not currently available in Canada

Main Side Effects

- Nausea and vomiting

- Fall in blood pressure with light-headedness

- Drowsiness

- Confusion/hallucinations

- Dyskinesia increase

- Constipation

- Sleep disturbances

- Daytime sleepiness with pramipexole

- Edema (leg and ankle swelling

Example of a Schedule for Starting Bromocriptine (Parlodel)

Continue all other medications as instructed by your doctor.

Bromocriptine 2.5 mg.

Take 1/2 tablet tonight with food.

Add 1/2 tablet every 3 days as explained below.

Day Number	Breakfast	Lunch	Dinner
1			1/2
3	1/2		1/2
6	1/2	1/2	1/2
9	1	1/2	1/2
12	1	1	1/2
15	1	1	1
18	1 1/2	1	1

Continue with this schedule until you are taking 2 tablets three times a day.

COMT Inhibitors

COMT (Catechol-O-Methyl Transferase) is an enzyme that helps in the breakdown of levodopa and is found both within the brain as well as in the peripheral nervous system (for example: nerves within the stomach). **COMT inhibitors such as entacapone (Comtan) and tolcapone (Tasmar) help prevent the enzyme COMT from breaking levodopa down**. Both of these drugs block COMT activity peripherally and tolcapone also has a mild central effect in the brain. **By blocking the activity of COMT there is an increase in levodopa availability to the brain**. They have no effect on their own if not used in conjunction with levodopa. Many studies have now shown that these drugs do prolong the availability and improve the response to individual doses of levodopa. Their **main indication is for patients who are having difficulty with motor fluctuations** (e.g. end of dose, wearing-off effects) but benefit has also been observed in non-fluctuating patients.

COMT inhibitors increase levodopa availability to the brain and are associated with an **increased incidence of levodopa side effects** (dyskinesia and less often confusion/hallucinations). Because of this, levodopa may have to be reduced by up to 30%. For patients who **already have a moderate amount of dyskinesia, the total levodopa daily dose should be decreased by 20 to 30%** at the time the COMT inhibitor is started. In general, the COMT inhibitors have few side effects, are easy to administer and have a rapid onset of action. The rapid onset of action means that if side effects like dyskinesia are going to develop they are normally seen within 24 to 48 hours after the medications are started. Therefore it is a good idea to start them early in the week (not on Friday) because if troubles arise it will be easier to contact your physician.

Tolcapone was the first of the COMT inhibitors to be approved. One of its uncommon side effects (1-3%) was an elevation of liver enzymes that if detected early, was felt to be reversible when the medication was stopped. This required that frequent liver function tests be done when the medication was first started. Unfortunately, three people have died as a result of sudden liver failure and this has resulted in the **medication being withdrawn from use in many countries**. It is still available in the United States but requires frequent liver function tests.

Entacapone has not been associated to date with any abnormalities of liver function and will likely be released for use in the near future. **Entacapone must be taken with each dose of levodopa** but tolcapone is taken three times a day, typically at six-hour intervals. Trials are underway with low dose Sinemet and a COMT inhibitor to see if the motor complications of levodopa are reduced.

Common Drug Name	Generic Drug Name	Daily Dosage (Milligrams)
Tasmar	tolcapone	300-600
Comtan	entacapone	400-2000

Main Side Effects

- dyskinesias

- hallucinations/confusion

- nausea

- diarrhea

- urine discoloration

- elevated liver enzymes (tolcapone only)

Monoamine Oxidase-B (MAO-B) Inhibitors (Selegiline-Deprenyl-Eldepryl)

Selegiline (Deprenyl) is a drug that acts **by inhibiting an enzyme** (MAO-B) which inactivates dopamine in the brain and in this way more dopamine is made available. Because of this effect, selegiline may give some relief of symptoms in newly diagnosed, very mildly affected patients, and may delay the need for levodopa for up to one year. When used without levodopa, selegiline has only a small effect on Parkinson's.

Selegiline is much more useful in patients at all stages of Parkinson's when combined with levodopa therapy (Sinemet or Prolopa) and may give relief of tremor and slowness. The drug also improves motor fluctuations in at least one half of levodopa treated patients however it may increase the chance of developing dyskinesias. It was initially hoped that selegiline would delay the progression of Parkinson's but **studies to date have shown minimal, if any, protective effect** (see below).

It also **causes a number of uncommon but serious side effects**. Confusion, hallucinations, increased dyskinesias and lowering of blood pressure (postural hypotension) are the most frequent of these. The incidence of side effects is increased in levodopa-treated patients. Special care must be used when giving selegiline to older patients and it **should not be used** in patients who have a history of confusion or hallucinations. It can lower blood pressure and cause episodes of unconsciousness. Rare patients have been troubled with chronic nausea that often clears with dose reduction but may require withdrawal. The drug should not be used in patients with a history of serious cardiac disease (angina) or bleeding from peptic ulcer. **The drug should not be used with Demerol** (Meperidine) **or with cold or sinus remedies** (ephedrine and selegiline together could raise blood pressure). **Caution is recommended when this medication is taken with any antidepressant medication** (tricyclic antidepressants, serotonin reuptake inhibitors). There is a potential interaction between antidepressant medication and selegiline although this may be more of a theoretical concern. If someone is on selegiline and becomes troubled by depression, the selegiline should be discontinued for a few weeks prior to the introduction of the antidepressant medication. If possible, selegiline should be stopped about 10 days before major surgery although no clear problems have been documented.

Selegiline is a very long lasting drug that causes chemical changes in the brain, which may persist for six to eight weeks after stopping the drug. It has become apparent that doses much smaller than the usual 5 mg. twice daily are very effective. **Patients who have side effects at the higher**

doses may still retain benefit with no side effects with doses as low as a half of a tablet (2.5 mg.) once daily or even one to three times per week. Overall this medication is normally well tolerated but insomnia may occur and it is better if selegiline is taken early in the day. When selegiline is added to levodopa-treated patients, a 10 to 30% reduction in levodopa may be required.

The DATATOP Study involving 800 patients with early, untreated Parkinson's, investigated the effectiveness of selegiline in delaying the progress of the disability. The patients were divided into four groups: selegiline; tocopherol (vitamin E); a combination of selegiline and vitamin E; and a placebo group. It was found that selegiline delayed the need for levodopa therapy in patients with early Parkinson's. However, there was no consensus if the need for levodopa therapy was delayed because selegiline protects against the dopamine producing neurons being lost or if it improves the symptoms of Parkinson's. Longer follow-up of these patients has demonstrated that **selegiline did not seem to have a protective effect and did not prevent the development of motor fluctuations and dyskinesias**. It did reduce the incidence of freezing developing. A few, more recent studies done with fewer patients continue to suggest that selegiline may have a mild protective effect, but again this is controversial. One study from the United Kingdom found a significantly higher mortality among patients treated with selegiline plus levodopa however many subsequent studies disagree with this finding. Vitamin E has no effect on the progression of Parkinson's.

Common Drug Name   Generic Drug Name   Daily
Dosage (Milligrams)

Common Drug Name	Generic Drug Name	Daily Dosage (Milligrams)
Eldepryl	selegiline HCl (5.0mg tablets)	2.5-10
Deprenyl		
Atapryl		
Carbex		

Main Side Effects

- heartburn/nausea

- insomnia

- dizziness

- dry mouth

- confusion/hallucinations

- dyskinesias

- postural hypotension

Amantadine

Amantadine was first developed as an antiviral agent but was discovered by chance to have antiparkinsonian effects. It provides **mild to modest improvement in about two thirds of early patients**. It helps in alleviating tremor, rigidity and bradykinesia and may smooth out the wearing-off effect. Often the long-term benefit of the drug only becomes apparent when an attempt is made to withdraw it, and as a result, symptoms worsen and rarely a severe confusional state develops.

Its exact mechanism of action is unclear. It may act by enhancing the release of dopamine or by blocking dopamine re-uptake. More recently, it has been recognized that amantadine may block the action of another chemical messenger called glutamate and this may be responsible for some or most of its anti-parkinsonian efficacy. **It has been suggested that long term amantadine use improves survival in Parkinson's patients**, possibly by this last mechanism. Recently it has also been shown to improve levodopa-induced dyskinesias (25% or more) in the later stages of the disease and that this effect can last more than two years.

Amantadine is easy to use and normally well tolerated with confusion, leg swelling, nausea, blurred vision and dry mouth being some of the side effects. **In patients with memory and thinking deficits it can increase confusion and therefore should not be used**. It is excreted by the kidneys and should be used in lower doses and with more caution in older patients and patients with impaired kidney function. If leg swelling is a problem, some benefit may still be gained by giving the drug on alternate days. If amantadine is going to be **stopped** it should be done **slowly** as neuroleptic malignant syndrome has been suggested as a possible risk of sudden withdrawal. In patients who are having difficulty with confusion and/or hallucinations, amantadine is one of the drugs that is commonly discontinued. However, in rare instances the withdrawal of it may increase confusion and cause paranoia, hallucinations and agitation. This state may only clear if the drug is restarted. **In confused older patients it is safest to slowly withdraw the drug over several weeks with reductions every three to four days.**

Endantadine

Common Drug Name	Generic Drug Name	Daily Dosage (Milligrams)
Symmetrel Endantadine	amantadine	100-300 (100mg capsules)

Main Side Effects

- confusion/hallucinations

- worsening of memory

- leg and ankle swelling

- red mottled skin colour change of the legs

- nausea

- dry eyes and mouth

- insomnia

Anticholinergics

Anticholinergic drugs have been used in the treatment of Parkinson's disease for decades, preceding the availability of levodopa therapy. **Their major effect is on tremor with little**

or no effect on slowness or stiffness. All of the anticholinergic drugs are similar in action, therefore there are few reasons for trying more than one drug. The most commonly used are trihexyphenidyl and benztropine. The mechanism of action for these drugs is by blocking the action of a chemical messenger called acetylcholine. The depletion of dopamine as seen in Parkinson's gives an imbalance between acetylcholine and dopamine, and by administering this type of drug a better balance can be obtained.

Anticholinergics are sometimes used in younger patients in whom tremor is the predominant feature but side effects are common (including thinking impairment) and often limit their use. **Anticholinergics are now being used much less often because of their tendency to slow memory and cause confusion**. They may also aggravate dyskinesias (involuntary movements). Drugs that work in the dopamine system (levodopa and dopamine agonists) relieve tremor as well as anticholinergics and in addition improve slowness and therefore are the preferred early use drugs. **Older patients should not take anticholinergics.** Anticholinergics may precipitate untreated glaucoma. Anticholinergics should be started and stopped very slowly over many weeks or months. Sudden withdrawal may markedly aggravate parkinsonism whereas very slow cautious withdrawal by 1/2 or 1/4 tablet reductions may hardly be noticed. Most experienced Parkinson's neurologists now seldom prescribe these drugs.

Common Drug Name	Generic Drug Name	Daily Dosage (Milligrams)
Artane	trihexyphenidyl	1-8
Cogentin	benztropine	0.5-8
Disipal	orphenadrine	150-400
Kemadrin	procyclidine	7.5-15
Paristan/Parsidol	ethopropazine	100-500

Main Side Effects

- blurred vision

- dry mouth

- constipation

- confusion/hallucinations

- memory slowing

- urinary retention

- impotence

- rapid heartbeat

- nausea/vomiting

Domperidone

Domperidone is a drug that is very useful for **reducing nausea and vomiting** and light-headedness on commencement of levodopa or dopamine agonist therapy. It is also **useful in**

increasing stomach emptying and decreases small bowel transit time and thus may improve levodopa absorption. Domperidone is best taken one hour before meals and usually has no side effects.

Common Drug Name	Generic Drug Name	Daily Dosage (Milligrams)
Motilium	domperidone (10mg tablets)	30-80

Main Side Effects

- dry mouth

- headache

Drugs for Essential Tremor (Propranolol, Primidone)

Many patients have very mild essential tremor and require no therapy once they are reassured that they do not have Parkinson's. Propranolol is a useful drug for managing essential tremor (see section on Essential Tremor). Propranolol has cardiac effects (it is a beta-blocker) and may slow heart rate and cause fainting.

Primidone may also help essential tremor. It has many side effects (nausea, sedation, headache) and must be started very slowly (62.5 mg. daily) to minimize them.

Common Drug Name	Generic Drug Name	Daily Dosage (Milligrams)
Mysoline	primidone (125mg tablets) (250mg tablets)	125-500

Main Side Effects

- reduced heart rate and fainting

- nausea

- diarrhea

- abdominal pain

- worsening of asthma (avoid use in asthma patients)

- depression

- fatigue

- impotence

Common Drug Name	Generic Drug Name	Daily Dosage (Milligrams)
Mysoline	primidone (125mg tablets) (250mg tablets)	125-500

Main Side Effects

- nausea

- heaache

- sedation

- blurred vision

Long Term Drug Adjustments for Parkinson's

If you are too slow, consider the following:

- More levodopa - a 50-100 mg increase in Sinemet one or several times daily may be all you need.

- Add another drug - Amantadine or a dopamine agonist or selegiline may help.

- Propranolol (see sections on Essential Tremor and Propranolol) may also relieve Parkinson's rest tremor (70% better in some patients).

- Observe the effect of high protein meals (see section on Weight Loss, Nutrition and the Low Protein Diet).

- All drugs should be reviewed especially any recent additions (see section on Drug Induced Parkinsonism).

- See section on Movement Problems.

Tips for Medication

- Use a pillbox (dosette) with separate compartments to store medications for a day; especially if going out. This helps to organize individual doses and avoids having to carry bottles. Prepare the day's drugs the night before or in the morning.

- Use a pill cutter. This can be bought from any drug store and is helpful in splitting pills for half or quarter tablet dosages.

- Keep medication at your bedside at night, especially if slow in the morning.

- Carry extra medication when going out, in case the trip takes longer than you anticipate. Take a day's supply of drugs.

- In case of emergency, carry a list of all your medication and dosages and the times these should be taken.

- **If confusion or hallucinations occur, all drugs for all conditions should be suspected and reviewed by your doctor.**

- Take medication after a light snack or meal. This reduces the side effects that may occur if taken on an empty stomach. If fluctuations are present it may be beneficial to avoid levodopa after a high protein meal. The ingestion of amino acids (which make up proteins) may slow absorption and may block the transport systems for levodopa entry into the brain (see section on Weight Loss, Nutrition and the Low Protein Diet). Many patients have no stomach problems with levodopa and can take it on an empty stomach. Patients with fluctuations should establish whether levodopa is more effective on a full or empty stomach.

- Chew Sinemet tablets for quicker onset of action (if necessary) except if nausea is a problem. Do not crush or chew Sinemet CR.

- Chronic mild nausea may be helped with a change to a levodopa compound with more carbidopa or benserazide. For example, change from Sinemet 100/10 to 100/25.

- Do not mix plain levodopa tablets and Sinemet. Marked short-term levodopa side effects may occur.

- It is quite reasonable for patients to adjust their levodopa (Sinemet or Prolopa) times (but not doses) to suit their own fluctuations and life patterns. Tell your doctor or clinic nurse of any changes on each visit.

- A mid-evening dose of levodopa may help on nights out.

- A very early morning dose of levodopa may help morning slowness or leg and foot cramps.

- If you are having vision or hand problems, ask your pharmacist for large print labels or non-child proof containers.

- Understand as much as you can about your medication. Ask regarding interactions with any new drug started.

- To improve your ability to swallow medications, take a sip of water to wet your mouth. Dip the tablets or capsules into water before placing them in your mouth. Follow the medication with a full glass of water.

- For patients with swallowing difficulties, place the medication on a spoonful of warm applesauce (see section on Swallowing Difficulty).

- Use one pharmacy for all your drugs. Get to know the pharmacist and discuss your drugs and interactions between them.

Note: Medication for Parkinson's is very individualized. You may have frequent changes in dosages and timing of your medication. Therefore your drug therapy may be very different from other patients. Improvement in mobility must often be weighed against drug side effects and many patients tolerate bothersome dyskinesias because of improved mobility. Hallucinations are so bothersome that patients and families will usually decrease levodopa and other drugs to clear them even if some mobility is lost (see section on Confusion and Hallucinations).

Over the Counter Drug Warning

Parkinson's patients should be careful in adding any new drug including ones your can purchase without a prescription (read the labels). For example:

- cough and cold remedies often contain antihistamines (Benadryl = diphenhydramine) which cause dry mouth and drowsiness

- decongestants (cough and cold) often contain pseudoephedrine or phenylpropanolamine (Robitussin CF and Primatene) and with selegiline or bromocriptine these drugs may induce high blood pressure and rapid heart rate

- dextromethorphan (Robitussin DM) occasionally causes dizziness, nausea, reduced blood pressure and rarely severe increase in temperature

- antacids and anti-ulcer drugs (Maalox or Mylanta) may increase levodopa (Sinemet) adverse effects. Also cimetidine or Tagamet may change body handling of drugs

Participation in Clinical Trails

This is a very worthwhile activity for patients to consider as their contribution to better treatment for Parkinson's. New therapies must be tested either against established ones or compared to no therapy (see section on Placebo Response). Often the patient and physician do not know which treatment the patient is on in a trial (called a double blind study). The studies are all reviewed and approved by an ethics committee (with lay representatives) before starting. The risks and benefits of the trial must be explained to you and you should eventually be informed of the study results.

Only after this careful process should a new treatment be accepted and in this way patients and their families can be given sound advice and reassurance that a new therapy has significant benefit.

The Placebo Response

The placebo effect is seen in all forms of treatment for human illness and is common in Parkinson's treatment. It does not mean that patients are being dishonest or trying to fool their doctor. **Some of the reasons are**: the patient wants to be better and also clinical trials involve extra visits, laboratory tests and personal contact with physicians and nurses. Some of the placebo benefits are not seen for up to six months. All the cardinal features of Parkinson's respond but bradykinesia shows the best improvement. Because of the placebo effect very small improvements with a new therapy are often viewed as not significant.

Alternative Therapy

The use of treatments outside the usual medication for Parkinson's is becoming more frequent and it is **important to understand why patients consider them. Some of the reasons are**: the desire to have hope, be well and do everything possible; the need to be involved in treatment decisions and to have control; the feeling that their treatment team is not looking after the "whole person"; and stress and strain caused by the diagnosis and difficulty in adapting to the limitations of the illness. Patients should discuss the use of complementary medicines with their doctor who should respond in a supportive way.

Parkinson's is associated with complex chemical upsets in the brain which are treated with drugs that are not perfect but have been carefully studied in the laboratory and tested in well controlled patient trials. **One must be very cautious in mixing into this delicate balance unproven and not well understood agents**. There is a report from eastern Canada of a child with leukemia who had a disease relapse after unproven remedies blocked a good chemotherapy result.

A few specific examples and cautions follow. St.John's Wort helps mild depression, it works in the serotonin system, the quality and dose are variable, side effects are few but a severe peripheral nerve upset on sun exposure has been reported. If you are depressed then discuss it with your doctor to be sure you are adequately treated. **Ginkgo Biloba** for memory impairment has been suggested but there is only a small amount of data to support this. It is a monoamine oxidase inhibitor and could induce the same side effects as selegiline (see section on Monoamine Oxidase B Inhibitors). It also blocks blood clotting and serious brain and eye bleeding have occurred in patients on aspirin and anticoagulants. **Melatonin** is used to induce sleep and is often helpful. It is also being studied as a treatment for sleep behaviour upsets (see section on Sleep) which is a complex chemical problem. This compound can block brain dopamine release and therefore must be used with caution in Parkinson's patients. The U.S. National Institutes of Health has developed a center to perform rigorous clinical trials to evaluate various unconventional treatments.

Chapter 3
Current Surgical Treatments

Surgical treatments for Parkinson's disease are not new and have been performed since the 1940's. However, with newer surgical techniques being available and the realization that medical management has limitations there is a renewed interest in surgical therapies. **Stereotactic surgical techniques are now used for**: the transplant-implant surgeries, lesioning procedures (permanent damage) and for the placement of deep brain stimulators. The transplant-implant procedures are still in the early experimental stages and therefore will not be discussed in this section (see section on Research and New Therapies). **Stereotactic surgery involves the use of needle probes**, which are guided to exact areas of the brain, using sophisticated computer and imaging (CT and MRI) systems. For some of the procedures, the surgeon also stimulates and/or records from cells as the probes are being inserted to help confirm that the desired location is found. In general, if patients are selected carefully, these techniques are of low risk and allow for the accurate location of the specific target that will give benefit.

There are currently **three main targets in the brain** for lesioning procedures or the placement of deep brain stimulators: **the thalamus, the globus pallidus and the subthalamic nucleus** (see diagram in section on Cause). With the improved understanding of the pathways or circuits in both normal and parkinsonian brains it has been learned that the above areas of the brain are **over active in Parkinson's patients. The surgeon may either make a lesion or insert a permanent probe to apply an electrical current** (deep brain stimulation) **at**

these locations to stop or decrease their function.

The probe is connected to a device similar to a heart pacemaker which supplies regular electrical pulses and must be programmed (see diagram).

At the tip of the stimulator probe there are four different contact sites that can be used to give the electrical currents. The ability to adjust the electrical

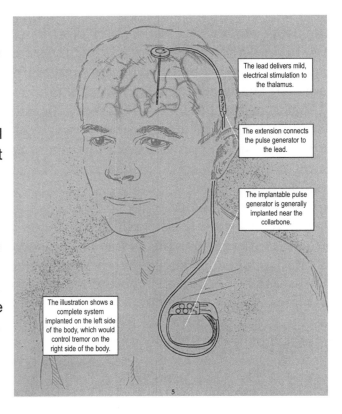

The lead delivers mild, electrical stimulation to the thalamus.

The extension connects the pulse generator to the lead.

The implantable pulse generator is generally implanted near the collarbone.

The illustration shows a complete system implanted on the left side of the body, which would control tremor on the right side of the body.

5

variables and/or change which contact site is being used gives a certain amount of flexibility to the deep brain stimulators, which may be beneficial in the long-term.

These procedures are performed while the patient is awake in the operating room, as the patient is required to give important information about eyesight, abnormal sensations and extra movements. They usually take between three and six hours to complete, making them very demanding on the patient. A successful procedure does not replace the need for medications in the majority of patients but instead **enhances the benefit from medical therapy and reduces medication side effects**. Not all patients are candidates for these procedures. Patients must realize that surgery is not a cure, nor does it affect the natural progression of the disease **but it can really improve function and quality of life**.

Lesioning Procedures

Surgical methods that destroy a part of the brain are called a **thalamotomy** if performed in the thalamus or **pallidotomy** if performed in the globus pallidus. A few patients have undergone stereotactic destructive lesions of the subthalamic nucleus (subthalamotomy) but there is a concern that this may cause extra abnormal movements (called ballism) and therefore it is currently not being performed in most centres.

Thalamotomy is one of the classical surgical treatments for Parkinson's disease. There are many different sub-regions within the thalamus but the specific region that is currently being targeted for treating tremor is called the ventral intermediate (Vim) nucleus of the thalamus (also known as the ventrolateral nucleus). **Thalamotomy is very effective in improving or completely relieving tremor in the majority of patients**. However it has little prolonged improvement in the other features of the disease (slowness or gait problems). The improvement in tremor is on the opposite side of the body to where the lesion is made in the thalamus. This is because most of the pathways that connect one side of the body to the brain actually cross to the opposite side (the right side of the body is controlled by the left half of the brain). If patients have severe tremor of both arms, then an operation is required on both sides of the brain. Recurrence of tremor occurs in up to 15% of patients, usually within the first three months. **Most patients with Parkinson's are not disabled from their tremor and therefore it is the minority of patients** who would be considered for this procedure but it can really improve function and quality of life.

Pallidotomy has its greatest benefit (>80%) in improving levodopa induced dyskinesia. A lesion is made in an area of the pallidum called the ventroposterolateral part of the internal segment of the globus pallidus (Gpi). The majority of the improvement on dyskinesia is on the side **opposite** the lesion and this seems to be a **long lasting effect** (four years plus). Some improvement is seen on the same side as the lesion but this improvement is usually temporary (one year). **Reduction of tremor, rigidity and bradykinesia are also seen, but the extent is more variable and the duration of benefit shorter than for dyskinesia**. Pallidotomy improves gait, freezing and postural stability but this effect is usually lost by six months. Pain associated with abnormal muscle spasms and rigidity is often almost totally abolished. Pallidotomy has a less consistent effect on tremor compared with thalamotomy. In general, pallidotomy can improve parkinsonian symptoms when patients are in their "off" phases but there is no improvement after surgery in patients best "on" function (except for the dyskinesias). This means that patients will not improve more than when they are in their best "on" phases with medication **but the length of time in this "on" phase is greater** (less fluctuations). For most patients their medication (levodopa) levels remain about the same following pallidotomy. However, because of better control of dyskinesia, some patients can tolerate higher doses of medication.

Both of the above procedures **are associated with potentially serious complications**. There is a 2-3 % chance of having a significant stroke (bleeding in the brain tissue) during the procedure with a less than 1% risk of death. **Speech and swallowing difficulties** occur in less than 10 % of patients who have a procedure performed on **one side only**, but there is a significantly increased risk (up to 30%) **when performed on both sides**. Difficulties with memory and thinking can worsen, again especially if bilateral procedures are performed. This is why patients with moderate or greater memory disturbances are not candidates for these operations. Significant weight gain has been reported in patients following pallidotomy. Persistent difficulty with vision used to be a problem following pallidotomy, however with improved surgical techniques this rarely occurs now. Other temporary side effects include: confusion, depression, facial weakness or a seizure (less than 3%).

Deep Brain Stimulation

Deep brain stimulation (DBS) for Parkinson's disease was introduced in the late 1980's for the treatment of tremor with the thalamus (Vim nucleus) as the target. The use of electrical stimulation does not mean that areas of the brain are "stimulated" to work better but instead **a high frequency current is given to stop the areas that are overactive from functioning. The risk associated with speech, swallowing or memory difficulties with bilateral stimulation procedures seem to be less than with bilateral lesioning techniques**. The intraoperative risk of causing a stroke is similar to that of the lesioning techniques being around 2%. Transient side effects are relatively frequent while programming is being performed and include; numbness, tingling, pulling sensations and double vision. **The major drawbacks of stimulation over a lesioning procedure are**: the implanted hardware could become infected (requiring that it be removed); the equipment fails or breaks; battery replacement (every three to five years for implanted devices); and the extra cost (~ $8,000 per stimulator).

Thalamic stimulation has now been shown to be highly effective in reducing tremor with benefit similar to that of a thalamotomy. If the stimulation is turned off the tremor rapidly returns. This effect on tremor in Parkinson's patients is sustained at least for a few years but for patients with essential tremor this improvement decreases with time. As for a thalamotomy, thalamic DBS does not improve the slowness or gait in Parkinson's but may have some effect on dyskinesias.

Fewer patients have had **chronic stimulation of the pallidum**. Pallidal stimulation, like pallidotomy, induces a dramatic effect on levodopa-induced abnormal movements but a variable effect on parkinsonian signs and symptoms. Some patients are greatly improved whereas others have only mild benefit. The programming of the stimulators can be difficult because some of the settings that result in the optimum control of dyskinesias may worsen slowness and seem to block the benefit derived from levodopa.

Stimulation of the subthalamic nucleus is evolving into the preferred target for Parkinson's patients. Tremor, stiffness and slowness are all clearly improved with this procedure and it may have long lasting improvement for gait and balance difficulties as well. There is a marked improvement in fluctuations with some patients no longer having any "off" time. It does not directly relieve levodopa-induced dyskinesias but because of the marked improvement in all the major parkinsonian symptoms, **levodopa doses can be drastically reduced and therefore the dyskinesias decrease.** In rare patients levodopa is stopped completely and patients remain fully mobile. Speech can be improved in some patients but not in others. Cognitive loss may be somewhat better with subthalamic nucleus stimulation (early report). No well-conducted clinical trials comparing pallidal to subthalamic stimulation have been performed but preliminary experience suggests that subthalamic stimulation has advantages over pallidal stimulation.

	Subthalamic Nucleus Stimulation	**Thalamus Stimulation or Lesion**	**Pallidal Stimulation or Lesion**
Tremor	+++	+++	++
Slowness	+++	0	+(+)
Stiffness	+++	+	++
Dyskinesias	++*	+	+++

The effects of stereotactic procedures on different targets:

+ = mildly effective;
++ = moderately effective;
+++ = greatly effective; 0 = no effect

* when the levodopa dose is reduced

Candidates for Surgical Procedures

As there is a risk of severe permanent complications with stereotactic surgery, only patients who are disabled, unable to cope with activities of daily living and require some assistance are considered. **All medical treatments that are possible should be tried first**. Patients should be otherwise in good general health, not depressed, not impaired cognitively, co-operative and severely disabled despite optimal trials of all available drug strategies and **still responsive to levodopa** (able to walk unassisted at least a few hours a day). Patients not considered candidates for surgical procedures include those with: severe heart, lung, kidney or liver disease; evolving cancer; moderate or greater difficulty with memory or thinking; severe depression; poor cooperation; and those able to cope with all activities of social or professional life without help.

Summary

- In carefully selected patients, surgical procedures can dramatically improve the lives of Parkinson's patients.

- The currently performed procedures are not a cure for the disease.

- The appropriate target is different depending on which symptoms are most disabling.

- A good result is more likely if the patient still has a good response to levodopa.

- The risk of side effects is small but serious ones do occur and therefore these procedures are only for patients who are disabled from their Parkinson's, despite optimum medical therapy.

Chapter 4
Research and New Therapies

In research lies hope for all who must live with chronic illness. This is the most exciting and optimistic time in history for brain research. The amazing pace of production of new knowledge, treatment concepts and novel therapies gives patients comfort, hope and optimism in their daily struggle. The advances being made in understanding basic mechanisms of cell function in many areas (for example cancer) give new tools for brain research. **It is becoming clear that many seemingly different brain diseases share some common mechanisms and new knowledge in one has relevance to another**. The mass of new understanding is the result of: coordinated effort; ease of scientific collaboration at a distance with new information technology; public and government research support; and the pharmaceutical industry who develop the new therapies for patient use.

It is now accepted that **not all the patient problems of Parkinson's are related to the loss of dopamine cells in the substantia nigra**. There are defects in other chemical systems (serotonin, cholinergic and noradrenergic) that play major roles in depression, thinking and sleeping. **The present focus of research effort is targeted at**:

• understanding the factors causing dopamine cell loss

• preventing progression

• early diagnosis even before symptoms and neuroprotection to avoid or delay the onset of the illness

- rescuing sick neurons, perhaps with growth factors

- developing new methods of drug and novel treatment delivery

- new surgical and transplant methods and materials

The following is a cross section of current research and potential new therapies.

New Methods of Delivery

Trials of a new dopamine agonist that is absorbed through the **skin** (uses a specific size skin patch) have been done. Drug delivery microchips (by mouth or absorbed through the skin) that release variable doses of multiple drugs are under study. Apomorphine (a fast acting dopamine agonist currently given by injection) preparations that can be taken by being sprayed into the nostrils or by being absorbed under the tongue (sublingual) have been studied. The nasal route has been found to be too irritating, however the sublingual method is effective and is better tolerated. Apomorphine use is complex with many side effects.

Levodopa ethylester is a new highly soluble oral levodopa solution for use in patients with disabling fluctuations and dyskinesias who are not controlled with standard regular or slow release levodopa preparations. There is now 10 years of experience using either slow constant, or intermittent, liquid levodopa preparations by mouth. These methods get around the slow stomach emptying and poor drug absorption seen in some Parkinson's patients (see section on Gastric Emptying).

Methionine

Methionine is an amino acid, which is used up in levodopa metabolism. **This depletion contributes to the long-term side effects of levodopa therapy**. Clinical trials are underway using dimethionine to replenish it and observe its effect in patients with levodopa related treatment complications

Lysoganglioside

Lysoganglioside is a semi synthetic derivative of GM1, which helped Parkinson's but required injection. GM1 is a trophic factor, which means that it is a chemical that can influence the development or repair of neurons. The original compound in its unpurified form had significant side effects. Lysoganglioside is active orally in laboratory animal models and shows promise. **The treatment concept is that these compounds may promote the development and repair of affected nerve cells and enhance the effect of natural body growth factors**.

Gene Therapy

Gene therapy is now being assessed in animal models of Parkinson's and human use is closer to reality. **The power of gene therapy lies in the capacity to use genes as drugs and to deliver genes, which control missing functions, to the brain by implantation surgery**. For example, the gene (tyrosine hydroxylase) that controls dopamine production is inserted into cells or viruses and implanted. New methods are being developed to give easier access to brain receptors by drugs and DNA (parts of genes).

Neuroprotection

Neuroprotection is the concept of slowing the progression of Parkinson's and eventually having treatments that stop Parkinson's from developing in the first place. There are multiple environmental and genetic factors that contribute to the basic cause of the illness but at present there is nothing definite enough to test as a complete prevention or protection agent. Oxidative stress is the best studied of a number of abnormal processes that contribute to the progression of Parkinson's once it has started. The **oxidation of dopamine** is a normal chemical process that becomes abnormal and produces toxic products that cause ongoing damage to dopamine neurons. Another process of dopamine cell loss in Parkinson's is a genetically controlled one called **apoptosis** or cell suicide. The steps in this are being understood and ways to alter them are developing.

It was hoped that selegiline, a monoamine oxidase-B inhibitor would slow this process but it has not clearly been demonstrated to do so. New drugs of this type are being tested including: transcyclopropine (blocks A+B types of monoamine oxidase) which has an increased blood pressure risk; and rasagaline a type B inhibitor. **The new brain scanning methods done early and during the protective treatment are being used as markers to try and show that these treatments truly prevent** dopamine cells from dying versus just helping the symptoms of the disease. (see section on Brain Scans).

Patient and family participation in these trials is critical in proving that new therapies truly slow or stop progression. The importance of clinical trials is shown by the selegiline story where there was **good laboratory** evidence that Parkinson's progression could be slowed. However, this beneficial effect was very indefinite **in human testing**.

Glutamate Antagonists

Glutamate is a neurotransmitter found in the brain. **Recent investigations suggest that a Parkinson's patient's brain may produce too much glutamate. Excessive glutamate overstimulates receptors leading to the death of neurons**. There are several types of drugs which can block the stimulation of the receptors and these are called **glutamate antagonists. It is felt that increased activity of glutamate (NMDA) receptors causes some late levodopa complications including fluctuations and dyskinesias** and may also contribute to disease progression. This is one of the ways amantadine works (see drug section on Amantadine). Rimantadine is a longer acting derivative of amantadine that is being studied. It has less side effects especially regarding confusion. Other drugs active in the glutamate system including budipine (Europe), dextromethorphan and novel experimental agents (remacemide, riluzole) that are being assessed. This is a whole new approach to restoring basal ganglia function and may be an alternative to surgery and should be tried before surgery is considered.

Stem Cells

The use of very primitive early cells called stem cells in human illnesses has generated great excitement. **The growth of these cells can be guided to produce very diverse kinds if tissues including heart, muscle or even dopamine producing brain tissue**. Work is now underway to identify the signals that tell a stem cell to become one tissue or another.

This will open new avenues for transplantation. There is also evidence that the adult human brain has some capacity to grow new cells and efforts now are to harness this potential into producing specific nerve cells that are deficient in human brain diseases like Parkinson's.

The above discussion is relevant for all the neurodegenerative illnesses and **shows how they are linked so that discoveries in one help understand another**. These links are obvious when one considers that some Alzheimer's patients develop features of parkinsonism and that the memory enhancing drugs developed for Alzheimer's may help some Parkinson's patients. This shows similar chemical problems in quite different brain illnesses.

Growth Factors

Growth factors have shown great promise in animal models of Parkinson's disease. Growth factors (GDNF) are now being directly injected into the fluid cavities of the human brain however the results to date have shown limited, if any benefit. **The concept is that these factors will "rescue" involved dopamine neurons, promote new connections and possibly increase survival of transplanted tissue**. The challenge in treatment is to develop methods to deliver these growth and "cell rescue" factors into the appropriate parts of the brainstem and basal ganglia.

By genetic manipulation, animal models of Parkinson's have been made. The Lewy body (the hallmark of the Parkinson's process) contains large amounts of alpha-synuclein, the gene defect found in some families (see section on Genetics). These animals overproduce alpha-synuclein.

These animal models (mice) will be critical in testing ways to interrupt this process and test other novel treatments.

Nurr1 is a molecule in brain that controls how much dopamine the brain makes. Mice with no Nurr1 are born with no brainstem dopamine neurons. Nurr1 seems to keep these cells active during life. One question is whether Nurr1 is affected by toxins and could we develop ways to keep it doing good things for dopamine neurons in Parkinson's patients.

There is excess iron in the brain of patients with Parkinson's. As well there are some abnormalities in body and brain handling of iron but this is not felt to be a primary factor in the cause of Parkinson's. No treatment suggestions have come out of the iron research work but each clue to the cause has to be studied.

Other Novel Therapies

Acupuncture

There has been one small study on acupuncture and it showed some very modest benefit in the "sit-walk-sit" test. This improvement in mobility was not accompanied by any change in detailed scoring scales. The treatment was twice per week for five weeks. It is questionable whether this is worth the effort and cost (see section on Placebo Effect) and it is probably better to invest the time and resources in other forms of therapy.

Transcranial Magnetic Stimulation (TMS)

Trials of this as treatment (done with coils over the head) have given no significant benefit. However research studies done using TMS to direct a magnetic field to temporarily disrupt the function of specific brain areas may give new understanding of brain function.

Tissue Implantation

Tissue transplantation into the brain (basal ganglia) for the treatment of Parkinson's has been an area of active research for many years. Since parkinsonism relates primarily to degeneration of the cells that make dopamine, attempts to **place dopamine-producing or dopamine-enhancing cells in the caudate nucleus and the putamen of the brain have been the focus of such studies.**

Adrenal to Brain Implants

Tissues from one of a patient's own adrenal glands were used. The results of a multi-centre study showed generally poor results without long term benefits.

Human Fetal Tissue Transplantation

Fetal tissue has been used in brain transplantation. Laboratory studies using human fetal dopamine tissue have shown functional improvement and host reinnervation. Transplants of human embryonic fetal brain cells into parkinsonians have been performed in many different countries with the best and most detailed results being from Sweden. A moderate degree of benefit from early studies has been obtained and a clear increase in basal ganglia dopamine has been shown.

A recent very detailed United States trial **showed modest benefit for younger patients (under 60) and the benefit was only in bradykinesia and rigidity**. There was no change in tremor, freezing, falls and walking. It is optimistic that there was some benefit but it is limited, complicated by some placebo effect, and **at present fetal cell implants in Parkinson's should be considered a research method that needs further study and improvement**. Agents that reduce the death rate of transplanted cells and also the use of growth factors with the implant are being studied. It is felt that immune suppression is not necessary.

Cell Culture Implantation

Using modern research techniques it is possible to produce and grow, non-fetal origin cells, that will benefit patients. **These cells can be modified to not only produce dopamine but also express growth factors** (see above sections on Gene Therapy, Stem Cells and Growth Factors). The patient's own skin or brain cells may be used. If cell culture implantation does become feasible, the moral complications of fetal tissue use are avoided.

Pig Tissue Transplantation

It has been shown that pig fetal dopamine cells will survive and make new connections when transplanted into human Parkinson's patients. There has been improvement with no evidence of viral infection, which was a concern. PET scans have not as yet shown increased dopamine production.

Carotid Body Cell Transplantation

The carotid body is a structure present on each side of our neck that helps determine the breathing rate by sensing the oxygen level in the blood. These cells are capable of making many times more dopamine then fetal cells and the cells survive much better then fetal cells. Results in animal models (rats, monkeys) show promising results and a patients own carotid body cells may be a good consideration as "donor cells" for injection into the putamen of patients with Parkinson's.

All of this shows the broad range of discovery and study now active in Parkinson's. We do not yet know why cells in the substantia nigra fail but we are clearly understanding the cascade of events that make it progress. This gives optimism and hope for patients in their daily struggle as they bravely carry on.

Disability With Advanced Parkinson's

The problems that disable patients with advanced disability include: postural instability and falls; increasing memory loss and drug induced confusion, hallucinations and personality changes; and disabling dyskinesias and motor fluctuations. The features that are present early in the disorder such as tremor and slowness continue to respond to levodopa. Walking, balance, voice, swallowing and bladder problems, which come on later in the disability, are less responsive to levodopa therapy.

Patients with severe disability should continue to be followed by Parkinson's clinics as many of the problems that develop can be relieved with various therapies. There is almost always something positive to do and this is often a great comfort to patients, caregivers and families. The major focus of this book and much of the research in Parkinson's is directed to relieving the problems of the more disabled patients.

On reviewing the following sections on common problems you will appreciate how many of the problems are related and linked together. For example: upset sleep is common to memory loss, depression, delirium, hallucinations and restless legs; and involvement of the nervous system outside the brain by the Parkinson's process results in problems with swallowing, speech, gastric emptying, constipation, bladder function, sweating, and low blood pressure.

Brain Tissue Donation

Leaving instructions that one's brain can be studied after death is a lasting contribution that the patient and family can make in the struggle to better understand the brain changes of Parkinson's. In this lies the hope for more precise therapies to improve treatment and prevent the onset of Parkinson's. **The original finding of brain dopamine that led to the development of levodopa therapy was made by the chemical analysis of donated brain tissue**. There is also a great need for normal brain tissue and families may consider this gift as well. The brain tissue banks cooperate and make tissue available to research groups worldwide. Pathologists and funeral directors are very respectful of family wishes and timelines and there should not be signficant additional costs. Your treatment team should be aware of your wishes and your physician and local Parkinson's society can help. If tissue is donated, a meeting with your neurologist to discuss and receive a copy of the results should be arranged. We have found this to be a very nice final review for the family and physician.

In Canada, contact:

The Canadian Brain Tissue Bank

The Bank 100 College Street, Suite 127

Toronto, Ontario

M5G 1L5

Canada

(416) 977 3398

There are similar tissue banks in the United States, the United Kingdom and most other countries.

Chapter 5
Common Problems and Tips to Overcome Them

Many of the problems experienced are caused by Parkinson's itself. Other problems are side effects of the medication. All patients do not experience all problems.

Handwriting

Difficulty with handwriting is one of the very early Parkinson symptoms. A patient's writing tends to become **smaller** as the symptoms appear. Tremor may also become noticeable in handwriting and many times the doctor will ask for a handwriting sample. Drug treatment for parkinsonian symptoms may improve writing but seldom brings it back to normal. There are special rubber grips available for pens and pencils, which make them larger and so, are easier to grasp. A felt pen may also be helpful. These devices are available at medical, stationary or school supply stores. Many patients use a typewriter, word processor or computer.

Memory Disorders and Emotional Problems

These disorders are extremely common and affect a large percentage of Parkinson's patients. They can be even more disabling than the motor difficulties. They may be part of the illness or result from its' treatment. **Serious cognitive impairment** (or dementia) **and delerium** (confusion) **are the leading cause of nursing home placement**. This group of problems is a source of much distress for the patient, family and caregiver and deserves careful evaluation. With attention to detail, very worthwhile treatment and relief are possible. **The

following problems will be discussed: cognitive impairment (with and without dementia); confusion and hallucinations; and behavioural impairments (including depression, anxiety, panic attacks and agitation).

Cognitive (Thinking) Impairment

It is estimated that up to 45% of patients with Parkinson's may have some impairment of thinking (cognitive) function. Of these, less than one half will be more severely affected (dementia). Mild impairment may not be recognized and the person just appears more passive and to have less energy. They deny depression, do not have guilt feelings, and usually do not respond to antidepressant medication. There will be some slowing of memory and information processing and the patient may not fully appreciate their problem. **These patients are at increased risk to develop confusion (delirium) with antiparkinsonian drugs**. Therapies used to treat early Parkinson's (anticholinergics or amantadine) can cause cognitive difficulty. Some of the new drugs for memory loss (donepezil or Aricept) are starting to be used for this mild impairment. For the majority of patients, mild memory loss will have little impact on activities of daily living and we must remember that mild impairment is common with increasing age. **More severe impairment (dementia) is a major problem and significantly changes the management of Parkinson's as drugs may easily induce confusion** (delirium). This degree of memory loss is seen more in: older patients; those with greater motor impairment; and those with a family history of memory problems. Dementia is uncommon in the first five years of the illness and if present early then the diagnosis may not be typical Parkinson's.

Great care with drugs is necessary as confusion and hallucinations are commonly induced and treatment of motor problems is more difficult and unsatisfactory because of this sensitivity to medication. There are several different brain processes to be considered in the patient with parkinsonism who has significant dementia. Typical Parkinson's does not seem to have a clear distinct pathological process associated with dementia, **rather in patients with significant memory difficulties, the final diagnosis may be either Alzheimer's disease, Diffuse Lewy body disease or Frontotemporal dementia.**

One third of **Alzheimer's patients** have signs of parkinsonism and this is a serious problem. These patients have more functional impairment than Alzheimer's alone and have rigidity and slowness with little or no tremor. There is an unusual loss of dopamine receptor sites in the basal ganglia (caudate and putamen) and this may explain the poor response of parkinsonism in Alzheimer's to levodopa.

Diffuse Lewy body disease is a common cause for dementia. The Lewy body is seen in the brainstem (substantia nigra) and is a major marker of Parkinson's. Some patients have these bodies all through the brain (cerebral cortex) and develop very distinctive signs. **They have visual hallucinations, fluctuating confusion, agitation, and parkinsonism**. The features of parkinsonism are seen early and are more prominent than in Alzheimers. They frequently have depression, increased daytime sleepiness and night upsets including muscle jerks and violent behaviour. The hallucinations and varying behaviour over the day are the hallmark of this problem. Rarely patients also have postural hypotension. Patients with Lewy body disease are extremely sensitive to neuroleptics (see below) and develop marked worsening of parkinsonism and require hospitalization.

Frontotemporal dementia is less common and patients may have profound personality change, poor social conduct, lack of motivation and insight. However memory may be fairly intact. Others have progressive speech difficulty (aphasia) with problems understanding but memory function is relatively preserved.

The cause of dementia is not clear and its' treatment is unsatisfactory. Nevertheless there have been major advances in recent years including greater understanding of the biology of cell changes in Alzheimer's and the importance of genetic factors. There are now animal models of Alzheimer's, that have given important new information. **The chemical abnormalities are being understood especially the reduced amounts of acetylcholine which can be improved** with specific drugs (donepezil and excelon) that stop it's breakdown. These drugs are effective in patients with mild to moderate impairment. Selegiline is not effective, and antioxidants (more potent than Vitamin E), estrogen replacement, anti-inflammatory drugs and nerve growth factors are being studied. Donepezil (Aricept) in low dosage has reduced **confusion, agitation and sleepiness in patients with Diffuse Lewy body disease**; higher doses may worsen parkinsonism (over 5 mg daily). Levodopa does not improve memory loss in Parkinson's.

Depression may at times be confused with memory loss and this should be carefully assessed, as depression is readily treatable.

Tips to Compensate for Memory Loss

- If you cannot recall a name or fact, relax and wait, there is a good chance that you will in a short time.

- Repeat a word or name several times to familiarize yourself with how that word or name sounds. This will greatly increase your ability to recall what it is you wanted to remember at a later date.

- When you are told something that you want to remember, connect the word to something that is meaningful to you. Usually a visual image is effective.

- Be relaxed. Feeling more relaxed allows the mind to be open to new information.

- Develop a routine where you always put something in a certain place and then you should always be able to find it.

- Carry a notebook to write down important items and date them.

- Avoid multiple pieces of paper with many notes.

- Keep a large kitchen calendar to note important events and appointments.

- Avoid situations where you have to make decisions rapidly, allow yourself time and request that people address you one at a time rather than having to attend to multiple people at any one time.

- Avoid demanding and stressful situations whenever possible and remind yourself that with a little time you will get there just as well.

Confusion and Hallucinations

This problem may be seen even before drugs are started but is most commonly treatment related. **If hallucinations develop early then the problem may not be typical Parkinson's**. This is often the first symptom of Diffuse Lewy body disease.

One of the most common (up to 1/3 of patients) late-stage treatment-limiting problems is drug-induced confusion and hallucinations. This is most likely to develop in memory impaired patients. The term **psychosis** is used if hallucinations and delusions are persistent. **Any of the drugs used in the treatment of Parkinson's may cause confusion, illusions or hallucinations**. Confusion may occur first and patients have difficulty with memory or reasoning. Perceptual changes may then develop and consist of illusions, in which objects may be mistaken for something else, and hallucinations in which non-existent people, animals or objects are seen. If the problem is severe then there may be manic behaviour, hypersexuality and paranoid psychosis.

Hallucinations are serious and unpleasant and require drug adjustment. This is the most common cause of nursing home placement. Hallucinations can affect any one of the senses including vision, smell, touch, taste and hearing. Visual hallucinations are most common. **As medication increases, the likelihood of hallucinations also increases**. When hallucinations become a serious problem, it may be necessary to either prescribe medication that specifically treats hallucinations or reduce the medication that is currently being given. Some patients experience the sensation of seeing unclear things at the side of their vision. This is also a drug effect but not as serious or upsetting as hallucinations and may not require a drug change. Some older patients with impaired vision have quite benign visual hallucinations.

Vivid dreaming or nightmares may be an early sign of levodopa induced problems. Later they can become more severe and frequent. Levodopa, dopamine agonists, anticholinergics, selegiline or amantadine may all cause these effects. The **worst offenders** are: drugs with major anticholinergic properties; selegiline, and dopamine agonists. Some patients may barely tolerate small amounts of levodopa. Almost any drug may worsen the confused parkinsonian patient. Pain medication, minor tranquilizers, antidepressants and drugs to reduce stomach acid have all caused problems. If the problem is of acute onset, the doctor may need to reduce the drugs significantly for a few days or a week and then use a lower dosage of the drug or stop one drug and change to another drug. In patients with advanced Parkinson's, the hallucinations or confusion are more difficult to control and **become a limiting factor in drug treatment**. Patients may accept mild confusion and illusions for better mobility.

There is a strong association between this problem and disturbed sleep. These patients waken frequently, they have altered dreams, night terrors and violent behaviour. The development of altered dreams is very significant and drug treatment should then be managed carefully.

Drug-induced confusion and hallucinations are reduced with the following therapy changes by your doctor:

• Withdraw anticholinergics or amantadine therapy (slowly if possible) as sudden stopping may worsen the problem

- Reduce or stop selegiline

- Stop a dopamine agonist

- Reduce levodopa - it is much safer to keep the patient on a small dose for a few days as stopping it completely requires hospitalization because of the risk of a severe, rigid, high fever, malignant hyperthermia-like illness

- Carefully review all other drugs for any condition

- Reduce bedtime antiparkinson drugs to help reduce mild night time upsets

- Pay attention to nutrition and fluid intake

- If the problem is severe and not improving then consider specific antipsychotic medication (see below)

A drug holiday is no longer recommended for the general management of late levodopa complications. Some very late-stage, memory impaired, drug-sensitive patients may be managed with only small, frequent, doses of levodopa-carbidopa.

There are a number of chemical factors that contribute to the problem of confusion including: excess stimulation of dopamine receptors throughout the brain, especially those concerned with emotion; overactivity of the serotonin system; and a reduction of cholinergic activity especially in older patients or those with memory loss (anticholinergic drugs therefore cause problems). From this, one can appreciate the basis for specific drug treatment. Drug treatment has become much better with our increased understanding of receptors and brain biochemistry.

The usual major tranquilizers such as haloperidol, block dopamine receptors throughout the brain, including the basal ganglia, and worsen **parkinsonism. Very specific drugs that just block dopamine receptors concerned with emotion** (and not motor function) **have been developed**.

Clozapine is available, however it causes drowsiness and **there is a risk of serious bone marrow depression** and at present weekly blood tests are required. Therefore it must be carefully monitored. **It usually does not worsen parkinsonism or thinking and is very effective in reducing dopamine induced delerium**. The usual starting dose is 12.5 (6.25 sometimes) mg at bedtime with slow increases. It also reduces anxiety, depression, hypersexuality, sleep disturbance and akathisia. In addition, tremor, dyskinesias, limb dystonia and pain show modest benefit. It may allow an increase in antiparkinson drugs after the delerium clears. Side effects include reduced blood pressure (first dose lying down), drowsiness, and high doses may cause seizures and increased saliva. It may be possible to reduce and stop it after a few months. As experience with the drug increases it seems safer than first thought and it should be seriously considered if other options have failed. New effective drugs with much less risk are now being used and developed.

Risperidone often increases parkinsonism and is not used frequently. **Olanzapine** helps about 50% of patients with psychosis and does not have the blood risks of clozapine. It may work best if the patient is just on levodopa and not on a dopamine agonist. It is most effective for psychosis caused by levodopa in patients who are not demented. Start in low dosage (2.5 -5 mg daily) at night to **avoid drowsiness**, which is the major side effect. It also reduces blood pressure and increases seizure risk. If the patient has been on clozapine then olanzapine is high risk for blood problems. It often increases parkinsonism and some patients have developed involuntary mouth movements (tardive dyskinesia). **Olanzapine has given variable results and has not been widely accepted by experienced Parkinson's specialists.**

Quetiapine (Seroquel) is a new drug of the same type. It has more attraction to serotonin rather than dopamine receptors and rarely increases parkinsonism. It does not have the blood concerns that clozapine has and is less likely to reduce blood pressure. It should be started in low dosage (12.5 - 25 mg daily) and if the patient is on clozapine the switch should be done with care. **Quetiapine has given excellent sustained results so far and may be the preferred drug for hallucinations and delerium caused by antiparkinson medication.**

Parkinson's patients respond to much lower doses of these drugs than are used in standard psychiatric care. **Ondansetron** (Zofran) is a serotonin blocking drug which has been very helpful especially for visual hallucination and paranoia. It is available (used for chemotherapy vomiting) but very expensive. New drugs of this type have been developed (granisetron) and studies are underway of cheaper agents that more easily cross into the brain.

Electro-convulsive therapy has also been helpful in improving severe hallucinations in non-memory impaired patients who do not respond to drug therapy or reduction.

Tips to Help the Family Cope With a Confused or Hallucinating Patient

- Remember this is almost surely a medication effect and this must be carefully reviewed.

- Make sure the patient is eating and drinking well. See section on in hospital care to avoid delerium.

- If the hallucinations are mild, explain to the patient that they are seeing things (bugs are common) that are not really there. Tell them the problem is caused by their medication. The patient will soon learn to recognize what is real and what is an hallucination

- Most mild illusions occur at night when shadows are misinterpreted as animals or people. Turn on more lights to reduce these shadows.

- When the patient wakes after a vivid dream or nightmare, turn on the lights. This will help them focus on reality.

- Some hallucinations and illusions are persistent but mild and not upsetting. Reassuring the patient does not stop the symptoms. They will insist that what they are seeing is real. Rather than causing constant friction, it may be better to avoid arguing.

- To move the hallucinating patient from their own familiar environment may cause an increase in the problem. Patients may be better in their own environment when drug adjustments to decrease hallucinations are being made.

- In rare cases, hallucinations may be extreme and

accompanied by delusions and paranoia. The patient may become agitated, aggressive or violent. Do not provoke. Do what is necessary to prevent injury. Call for medical assistance or 911 if necessary. Reducing anti-parkinson medication will always decrease symptoms.

Behavioural Impairments (Depression, Anxiety, Panic Attacks and Agitation)

Depression

More significant depression seems to be seen more in patients with memory impairment and greater disability, but it may even precede the onset of clinical parkinsonism. It may be related to a defect in serotonin metabolism. **Depression may be a major factor in the lack of response to antiparkinsonian therapy**. Sometimes, the clue is that the physician observes clear functional improvement, which the patient denies.

Common indications that a Parkinson's patient may be experiencing depression include:

• Worsened sleep with early morning wakening

• A decrease in memory

• A decrease in appetite, although older patients may eat more

• More bradykinesia and gait upset

• Loss of energy and interest; sadness, crying

• Feelings of guilt and helplessness worsened by recent retirement

There are two common types of depression that occur: **apathetic** (withdrawn) **and agitated**. The first treatment should be an attempt at counseling. If this fails then specific drug treatment is started. If the patient is **apathetic** then use selective serotonin reuptake inhibitors (SSRI's) as these have an activating effect. The drugs used are; fluovoxamine, paroxetine and sertraline. These drugs should not be used with selegiline (a rare bad serotonin reaction may result) and occasionally worsen Parkinson's and this should be watched for.

If the patient is **agitated** then tricyclic antidepressants are used as they have sedative effects. They do not worsen Parkinson's but because of their anticholinergic effects are more likely to induce delerium especially in memory impaired patients and may aggravate postural hypotension.

Drug treatment of Parkinson's patients with depression is usually for 6 to 8 months but can often be long term. **Electro-convulsive therapy** (ECT) is proving to be very helpful for depressed Parkinsonians without memory loss. In patients with significant thinking impairment, confusion and increased memory problems may be associated with ECT. Light therapy is also proving useful. **Depression is common, it is very treatable, and should be watched for and treated optimistically by the patient, family and treatment team.**

Anxiety and Panic Attacks

About 40% of Parkinson's patients experience anxiety with or without panic attacks. The panic spells are associated with dizziness, shortness of breath and sweating. These symptoms should be managed with short acting minor tranquillizers such as alprazolam, lorazepam or clonazepam. If the patient is not responding then watch for agitated depression.

Agitation

This can be induced by antiparkinson drugs or can be a reaction to Parkinson's. It is more common in memory impaired patients. Its treatment may require reduction of antiparkinson drugs and the use of minor tranquilizers and again agitated depression should be watched for.

Note: Any of these behavioural upsets may be seen during the off spells associated with motor fluctuations and will respond to adjustment of antiparkinson therapy.

Sleep Problems

Poor sleep is very common in Parkinson's. **It may affect up to two-thirds of patients and may be related either to the illness or its' treatment**. Poor sleep is common as we get older (sometimes it is a lifelong problem) but Parkinson's is associated with a whole new set of nighttime problems. Careful review with the patient and family is necessary to clarify the exact type of sleep upset and very worthwhile treatments are available. More sleep upset occurs with more advanced Parkinson's, long-term levodopa use, depression and cognitive problems. Bad dreams, muscle jerks, crying out and dyskinesias, all from excess levodopa may be a major component. Increased parkinsonism with pain, difficulty turning, frequent urination, cramps and muscle stiffness needs to be clarified and treated.

A variety of neurochemical defects contribute to sleep upset. These include reduced dopamine giving motor problems and serotonin deficiency causing depression and sleep cycle disruption. **The specific sleep problems that will be reviewed include**: insomnia, increased daytime sleepiness, upsets during sleep (including sleep violence), sleep benefit, morning worsening and restless leg syndrome.

Insomnia

The common pattern for insomnia is: wakening a few hours after falling asleep; being awake for a significant time; and then multiple more wakenings. The patient should be questioned carefully about wearing off episodes and increased parkinsonism causing difficulty turning, discomfort or frequent urination. Nightmares may add to the problem (see upsets during sleep). **Insomnia is a frequent symptom of depression and responds well to treatment** (see section on Depression). If the problem is anxiety or caused by a transient life upset then the use of a short acting minor tranquilizer like clonazepam or temazepam for short periods of time may be of benefit.

Tips for Insomnia

Review these and note the ones that relate to you.

• The pattern of sleep must be reviewed in detail.

• Define any nighttime Parkinson's problems including nightmares.

• If dyskinesias are a problem, then reduce levodopa at bedtime.

- Wearing off may require a late dose of slow release Sinemet or a dopamine agonist.

- Selegiline may worsen sleep, Amantadine is occasionally a factor.

- Establish whether depression or memory loss are significant factors.

- Do not go to bed too early.

- Avoid alcohol in the evening.

- Avoid bedtime dose of levodopa if possible if nightmares are a problem.

- Become more socially active during the daytime.

- Develop a bedtime ritual as it will remind your body that it is time to go to bed.

- Drink warm milk before bedtime.

- Your doctor may prescribe a light sedative, for example Lorazepam (Ativan), or Oxazepam (Serax).

- Before going to bed try and make sure you are relaxed and tired. Being generally stressed or worried about how much sleep you are going to get that night will only keep you awake.

- Exercise regularly, but not right before going to bed.

- Establish a regular schedule of going to bed and getting up. Set your alarm clock for a certain time every morning and wake up at that time no matter how much sleep you got that night. A consistent routine like this will establish a sleep cycle for your body.

- Get plenty of bright light during the day and try not to spend a lot of time in bed during the day.

- Daytime naps are fine especially if overnight sleep is poor. As sleep improves try and make them shorter.

- Avoid caffeine in the evening.

- Take a warm bath and perhaps read part of a good book before sleeping.

- Satin sheets may help turning in bed; be careful near the edge of the bed.

- A diaper system or condom catheter may be needed if urinary frequency is not controlled with medication.

- Avoid eating a large meal before going to bed.

- If after being in bed awhile and still unable to sleep, get out of bed and read or watch television for awhile. Trying to force yourself to sleep only further wakens you.

- Learn relaxation exercises and use them as you settle for sleep.

Increased Daytime Sleepiness

Fatigue may be a major problem simply related to a poor overnight sleep. One of the major causes is medication and especially levodopa. Anti-anxiety drugs taken at night or during the day will contribute. It becomes worse with increasing doses. This is difficult to treat. Slow release Sinemet may worsen this and a dopamine agonist combined with levodopa reduction may help. However the new dopmaine agonist, pramipexole may itself cause daytime sleepiness (see section on Dopamine Agonists). Depression causing insomnia should be watched for and treated with an antidepressant that has alerting properties (see section on Depression). Stimulants (amphetamines) are not useful and taking levodopa only on alternate days will give much less sleepiness on the "no-dose day." A slightly higher than regular dose may be needed on the "dose day."

Tips for Daytime Sleepiness

• Increase the daily amount of caffeine intake.

• Plan a regular routine of exercise, about five to ten minutes two or three times daily.

• Decrease the amount of Sinemet at each dose.

• Consider a dopamine agonist (watch pramipexole) and reduce Sinemet.

• Taking Sinemet on alternate days occasionally helps.

• Some other medical problems such as low thyroid function may be an unrecognized treatable factor.

• Daytime sleepiness may also be the result of boredom, lack of social activities or depression. Try to become more active, if not physically, then mentally. Admit to feelings of depression and seek medical advice.

Upsets During Sleep

Upsetting dreams and talking and walking during sleep may **all be signs that the dose of levodopa is near its' upper limit**. Various muscle jerks may occur during sleep and these are related to levodopa. They usually do not waken the patient but may upset the bed partner. Tricyclic antidepressants (amitriptyline) may increase nighttime movements and behaviour upsets.

Sleep violence occurs in up to 15% of treated Parkinson's patients. It involves nocturnal kicking, running, punching, thrashing and pushing. Partner's often report injury and if wakened, patients report bad dreams. This sleep upset is called REM (Rapid Eye Movement) sleep behaviour disorder. This should be reported to the clinic team and a thorough review of all drugs done. If medication reduction is not helpful or possible then clonazepam usually helps (see section on Hallucinations).

Sleep Benefit

Up to 50% of Parkinson's patients report improved motor function and feeling better in the morning. This may last one to three hours and many patients are able to delay their first dose of medication. Patients who note this tend to be older, male, have more night wakenings, and have had Parkinson's for a longer time. They do not have more nightmares, hallucinations or sleep violence. There is no relation between taking a bedtime slow release Sinemet and morning sleep benefit. These patients insist that this is their best time of the day.

Morning Worse

The opposite of sleep benefit is also seen, some patients are worse on wakening. They usually keep Sinemet by their bed to achieve first mobility. A night dose of a dopamine agonist may help.

Restless Leg Syndrome

This is an irresistible desire to move the legs or to walk. It is associated with numbness, aches and cramps. These patients also have delayed sleep onset and multiple wakenings. **This is very common in Parkinson's but is also seen in 10% of the population**. It occurs in the day but is markedly worse at night either before or during sleep. If severe it is very upsetting to the patient, seriously disrupts sleep, and causes sleep deficiency and daytime drowsiness. It can cause major problems in home, social and work life.

The cause of restless leg syndrome is not clear and must be differentiated from levodopa-induced dyskinesias and akathisia. Recent PET studies have shown reduced basal ganglia dopamine function. Treatment is complex with variable results, which often do not last. Levodopa helps but Parkinson's patients are usually on it already (slow release Sinemet sometimes is of benefit). However with levodopa the duration of benefit shortens, end of dose rebound worsening occurs and previous nighttime only symptoms can become problematic during the day. **Dopamine agonists frequently give relief and the newer agonists, pramipexole and ropinirole have shown excellent sustained benefit in initial trials and may be the preferred treatment**. Patients report better sleep, reduced leg sensory symptoms and leg discomfort. This is achieved with very low doses of pramipexole (0.5 to 1.0 mg). Clonazepam often helps. Codeine in small doses may be tried as a last resort but there is concern about addiction and it may upset sleep on it's own. As always, watch for a component of drug induced dyskinesias. Tricyclic antidepressants may worsen restless leg syndrome.

Leg Cramps

Leg cramps may affect people without Parkinson's and **are a very frequent and upsetting problem in parkinsonism and cause major sleep disruption**. The patient usually is wakened with severe calf or foot pain, which is often prolonged. The pattern may vary over weeks and months. A number of other medical conditions may also cause cramps. These include: low thyroid function; low potassium (usually related to diuretic or water pill use); and lumbar disc disease with single or multiple nerve irritation. Blood vessel problems in addition to the just noted disc troubles, are more likely to cause pain and cramps on walking. Disc related walking pain has been reported to be helped with increased levodopa.

Tips for Leg Cramps

- Do nightly calf stretching exercises. These may be the most helpful preventives. Stand two feet from a wall, lean forward against it keeping your feet flat on the floor, hold and repeat. These could be also be done in bed for the patient.

- Sleep under loose covers to avoid pressure on your toes. A pillow at the end of the bed may also help.

- If a cramp occurs either: straighten the whole leg out and bring the foot back up toward the knee; or grab your toes and pull upward. Massage the muscles in spasm. Heat may help.

- Slow release Sinemet or a dopamine agonist at bedtime may help. It may be important to clarify if dyskinesias (needing drug reduction) are a component.

- Minor tranquilizers (lorazepam), or carbamazepine (used for seizures) may help. Quinine (another tranquilizer) should not be used as its' help is minimal and there are serious side effects (rash, cardiac, vision).

- Morning cramps and dystonia will improve with a dose of Sinemet taken on wakening (chew one half of a 100mg tablet and wait 30 minutes before rising); keep the dose on your bedside table.

Cramps, like dyskinesias may slowly decrease over time. One of our severely disabled patients was given small doses of morphine a few times a week for 3 months and cramps cleared completely.

Fatigue

Fatigue is a common symptom in Parkinson's (30 to 40% of patients). It may be a very prominent and disabling complaint and it is not always associated with more severe disability, sleep disturbance or medication effect. It is seen even in mildly disabled patients. There is much discussion as to whether fatigue is of muscle (mitochondria) or brain (dopamine deficiency) origin. Studies in Parkinson's patients have clearly shown that a dose of Sinemet will significantly reduce fatigue. Detailed muscle strength assessments have shown that the side most involved with Parkinson's improves best. **This levodopa response suggests that brain dopamine deficiency is a major component.**

Fatigue is more common with depression but many non-depressed patients have bothersome fatigue. It is difficult to treat and response to antidepressants and stimulants is variable. **An exercise program** should be tried to improve conditioning; especially since it has been shown that Parkinson's patients may be somewhat energy inefficient and have to work harder for adequate oxygen exchange and tissue metabolism.

Frequent tremor or abnormal involuntary movements may also cause fatigue. Normal everyday activities require more time and increased effort to complete. **To help overcome these problems**, plan your day activities carefully. Give yourself more time to complete them. Pace yourself and include daily rest periods. Plan special activities to occur at the time of day when your medications are most effective. Make use of the many products available to help reduce the effort for routine activities (see section on Assistive Devices and Techniques).

Patients note that Parkinson's fatigue is different than the fatigue experienced before the illness began. This and the levodopa response are arguments against depression as a major factor and indicate that the **best relief from fatigue will come with optimum adjustment of antiparkinson medication**.

Bladder Problems

Difficulties with urination are part of Parkinson's and affect up to 40% of patients. The first symptom is usually frequent urination at night (nocturia) and often a sensation of incomplete bladder emptying is noted. Also a sense of urgency develops. If daytime frequency and urgency precede the night frequency then the problem may be a flow obstruction such as prostate enlargement. If there is any worsening of symptoms, even if there is no discomfort, then a urine culture should be done as infection is common with incomplete bladder emptying. **In most patients, bladder dysfunction is mild and more of a nuisance** however for some patients it is a major personal and social problem. Some patients have urinary frequency during off periods and this may add to overnight problems. Some patients, and especially those with non-typical parkinsonism have much more urinary difficulty. In these patients, urgency and frequency are worse and incontinence of urine is common. For these patients urgency is overwhelming and incontinence results.

Drugs used in the treatment of Parkinson's may alter bladder function. Rare cases of bladder upset have been reported with levodopa or bromocriptine and drugs with anticholinergic activity (trihexiphenidyl or amitriptyline) tend to slow bladder function and rarely, may cause retention (inability to empty bladder). **Bladder specific anticholinergic drugs** (Ditropan = Oxybutynin chloride) are often **most helpful in treating urgency and frequency**. These drugs still have some risk of inducing confusion, as do all anticholinergics (see section on Anticholinergic side effects). A new anticholinergic (Detrol or tolterodine) has just been released and gives less dry mouth than Ditropan. In addition dopamine agonists (pergolide studied the most for this) may markedly reduce urgency, frequency and incontinence. Because of their similar nerve supply, bladder and sexual problems may occur in the same patient.

Tips for Bladder Problems

- If bladder problems are bothersome, see a urologist, and if possible see one with a particular interest in neurological difficulties. This is important to assess any element of obstruction (prostate or narrowed urethra) which might be helped by surgical treatment or dilatation. The trend now is away from surgery for benign prostate enlargement and more conservative treatments (including drugs) are favored.

- Females may have incontinence on straining from bladder changes secondary to childbirth. A urologist or gynecologist should be seen.

- Bladder infections should always be considered and can be diagnosed by your doctor ordering a urine culture.

- Limit fluids after dinner or if going out. This avoids nighttime problems or embarrassing situations.

- Reduce consumption of drinks which have a diuretic effect (causes urine to be formed and released) for example; coffee, tea, grapefruit juice or soft drinks containing caffeine. Patients are often on water pills (diuretics) for high blood pressure or leg swelling and these will worsen urgency, frequency and incontinence.

- Exercise pelvic muscles to increase retention of urine. Control can be improved by starting and then halting the flow of urine.

- If incontinent, you may be more comfortable using cotton underwear with liners or disposable pads. Immobility or slowness to get to the bathroom may cause nighttime incontinence. Keep a urinal, bedpan or commode nearby. Men may wear a condom catheter if lack of bladder control causes wetting.

- Drinking cranberry juice can be helpful in reducing the unpleasant odours associated with bed wetting or soiling of clothing. There is also some recent evidence that it may prevent recurring urinary infections.

- Levodopa may occasionally cause a reddish brown stain in urine. This may occur on underwear or toilet bowl water that has been washed with bleach (alkali). Tests should be done to exclude bleeding.

- Better treatment of motor fluctuations may reduce off period urinary frequency. Consider this at night and overnight levodopa may help and also dopamine agonists have proven very helpful.

- Specific drug therapy for bladder problems (for example Ditropan or Detrol or the antidepressant imipramine) is often remarkably helpful. In the past many patients had good relief with Ditropan and Detrol is now worth a try especially if dry mouth is a problem with Ditropan. The two drugs have almost the same bladder effect. In men Finasteride (Proscar), an enzyme inhibitor has been found to be effective, as it reduces the production of androgen and decreases the size of the prostate.

- Incontinence demands a full urological assessment as treatable causes are frequently found.

Sexual Problems

Most sexual problems in Parkinson's are related to the illness itself. This is very common and 40 to 60% of patients are affected to some degree. Sexual function decreases with age and this can be accelerated up to six times in patients with chronic illnesses such as Parkinson's. The need for intimacy and sexual expression are significant components of quality of life and should be discussed with patients. **Much can be done**. Physical limitations including tremor, slowness and reduced coordination add to the problem and stiffness and tremor may increase with arousal and orgasm. Sexual dysfunction may be further aggravated by depression, which is also part of the illness and also anxiety and frustration. In men, the most common problem is difficulty in producing and maintaining an erection. In men and women, a decrease in interest in sexual activity and orgasmic function is common. A reduction in libido has been noted even in young patients. A recent study of sexuality in women with Parkinson's showed that there was often dissatisfaction with the quality of the sexual experience and with their partners. Many report changed orgasms with a number of high points and an abrupt stop. Anxiety, inhibition, vaginal tightness and fear of incontinence are also contributing factors in inhibiting sexual motivation.

There should be a thorough medical evaluation. Postural hypotension (see below) and urine and fecal control problems may indicate more widespread nervous system malfunction. Hormone levels including prolactin should be checked in males and females. Depression is common and needs review.

Getting proper help often requires some innovation especially for females. Men are referred to urologists who often have specialized clinics. For women it is worth checking if they can help especially if there are bladder symptoms. Discuss with your family doctor or gynecologist. There are few physicians who are declared sexual medicine consultants and your help may be a combination of your clinic team, family physician, gynecologist and urologist. Specialty clinics often have long waits - persevere.

Many drugs used for other conditions can decrease sexual function and this should be carefully reviewed. Common problem ones include: codeine, thiazide diuretics, selective serotonin reuptake inhibitors (60% of patients) and tricyclics (desipramine safest) for depression, cimetidine, drugs for anxiety (lorazepam safest), beta blockers (for tremor or hypertension) and monoamine oxidase inhibitors. As noted above, depression is common as a contributing factor and treatment must be carefully chosen. Some of the new cardiac and antihypertensive drugs have sexual adverse effects. The effect of antiparkinsonian drugs is variable; levodopa or dopamine agonists may give minimal improvement in sexual function in some patients. Occasionally, patients may have a marked increase in sexual function with levodopa, dopamine agonists and other drugs and this may be accompanied by very inappropriate behaviour. This increase suggests that a lack of dopamine is a component but the problem is much more than this and antiparkinsonian drugs should not be increased for sexual dysfunction. The bothersome increase may occur at times of peak drug effect and usually improves with dose reduction. Many illnesses and medications that impair penile and clitoral blood supply reduce sexual activity and many of these problems are felt to be related to lack of proper blood supply.

Sexual function is an important part of human relationships and problems should, and frequently can, be treated. If your treatment team does not ask then raise your concerns - it is part of the illness.

Drug Treatment for Sexual Dysfunction

Sildenafil (Viagra)

Normal erection depends on relaxation of smooth muscle and Viagra works this way in response to sexual stimulation. The dose is 25 to 100 mg taken one half to four (usually one) hours before. A recent study of male Parkinson's patients reported excellent results with minimal side effects (facial flushing is most common) with a 50 mg dose and studies are underway with female patients. If **you are on nitrates (for angina) you should not use Viagra** as a major drop in blood pressure may occur. If you have postural hypotension with Parkinson's then be careful, as a ten-point drop with the drug is common in non-affected persons. Headaches may result. Transient blurred vision occurs and if you have retinal disease then discuss this with your eye doctor.

Alprostadil and Muse

These agents are injected into the urethra of males and give much less whole body side effects. They act immediately but are awkward and occasionally cause some penile pain.

Tips for Sexual Problems

- Decreased sexual function does not mean decreased love for the partner.

- Understanding and patience are helpful.

- Changes in antiparkinsonian drug therapy rarely will improve erectile function.

- Other drugs for other problems (such as high blood pressure or anxiety) may contribute to sexual problems (see above).

- Seek help and treatment as outlined above.

- Treatment for depression may give benefit. The right drug must be selected, as some will worsen sexual function.

- Antiparkinson medication can sometimes cause an abnormal increased interest in sexual activity. If this occurs, the patient or family member should inform the physician so that appropriate medication changes can be made.

- Sexual activity should be regular. Inactivity reduces oxygen supply and erectile function.

- Have an open discussion with your partner. Try to understand each other's difficulties and needs and find ways to solve them.

- Chronic illness is tough on both of you. So relax, think positive, and enjoy and share each others love in whatever ways you can.

- Menopausal problems need to be addressed.

- Insist on a full workup for problems unrelated to Parkinson's that may be contributing to sexual dysfunction.

Postural Hypotension

Postural hypotension **is a drop in the patient's blood pressure** which usually occurs when changing position, for example, rising from a chair, getting out of bed or bending over. It may also occur a few minutes after standing. The diagnosis is made when there is a 20 point systolic drop or 10 point diastolic drop.

The problem is caused by **involvement** (by the Lewy body Parkinson's process) **of the central and peripheral nervous systems that control blood pressure**. In addition similar changes have been described in the nerve supply of the heart. Lightheadedness or faintness is experienced and is sometimes accompanied by transient visual loss, loss of consciousness, multiple falls and serious injury. It can cause unsteadiness walking which improves with higher blood pressure.

Factors that contribute at any one time are: food, time of day, state of hydration, temperature, recent lying down and medication. Treatment is considered only if there are symptoms. A pattern must be established as blood pressure and symptoms vary over the day. **Postural hypotension is made worse by levodopa, dopamine agonists, selegiline, anticholinergics and antidepressants with strong anticholinergic effects** (amitriptyline is one). Domperidone gives improvement in a few patients. Some patients with atypical or severe parkinsonism may have a major problem with postural hypotension. For many patients the quality of life may be significantly improved by reducing postural hypotension.

Three Approaches to Treatment of Postural Hypertension

- **Increase the fluid volume in blood vessels**. Florinef, a salt retaining steroid or increased salt are used. A response to Florinef is seen within one week. Dose increases are necessary and side effects are foot and leg swelling, a five to seven pound weight gain and with long term use cataracts and osteoporosis may occur. Indomethacin (used for arthritis) is sometimes combined with Florinef, it is stomach irritating.

Caution is needed as this gives much fluid retention. Florinef lowers blood potassium and this should be checked and extra potassium taken in the diet (dates, prunes, nuts, bran, tomatoes, potatoes).

- **Improve peripheral blood vessel resistance**. The drugs used are Ephedrine or Midodrine. The dose of Ephedrine is 30 mg one to four times daily. Midodrine dose is 2.5 mg taken before breakfast and lunch and mid afternoon. It should not be given at bedtime (may cause hypertension when lying) and the maximum daily dose is 10 mg. Midodrine works within hours and may be good for blood pressure drops in the morning and after meals. It may be combined with Florinef and the dose of Florinef can be reduced.

- **Correct anemia (low blood count)**. If anemia is present it is treated with erythropoetin injections twice weekly for six weeks.

Tips for Postural Hypotension

- All drugs should be reviewed. Blood pressure tends to slowly decrease over the years in Parkinson's and a previous diuretic (water pill) or other high blood pressure treatment, **can often be stopped**. Many cardiac drugs lower blood pressure. Levodopa in combination with carbidopa (Sinemet) has a less hypotensive effect than levodopa only.

- Check for anemia, it is common and treatable.

- Keep the head of the bed elevated (14 degrees) at night with a pillow or blocks secured under the legs of the headboard. Patients should be instructed **not to lie flat even in the**

daytime as this increases blood pressure, salt and fluid loss making postural hypotension worse especially in the morning. Also a carbohydrate snack or exercise at bedtime will reduce lying blood pressure in the first few hours of sleep.

- Drink more fluids. Water drinking will significantly raise seated and standing blood pressure. The response occurs in five minutes, reaches a maximum in 30 minutes and persists for one hour. It is very useful in the morning before drugs take effect. Be careful lying down after water as a dangerous increase in blood pressure can occur.

- Avoid standing in one place too long. When standing, rock from one leg to another or squeeze the legs together, raise the toes, put one leg up on a chair, all to tighten the leg and thigh muscles. This stops blood from pooling in the legs.

- **If you feel faint raise your arms over your head for 15 seconds**. Some blood drains down but more importantly the heart pumps blood to the brain because the arms are higher. This is a new idea, it is reported to give instant results. You will be aware of the radial pulses at the wrists.

- Sit down as soon as you feel faint.

- Elastic or support stockings may be of use if they cover the thigh as well as the calf. They are not comfortable or popular or very effective. A well fitted abdominal binder may help and must be put on in the morning.

- Be more careful of drops in blood pressure **after meals and on warm days.**

- Eating small meals with caffeinated beverages may alleviate drops in blood pressure. The smaller meals may help to prevent blood pressure drops, which can occur after large meals when much blood goes to the stomach. As well, the caffeine constricts blood vessels, which can avoid blood pressure drops.

- Avoid taking hot showers, using alcohol and excessive exercise, if postural hypotension is experienced frequently.

- Increase your salt intake by adding more table salt to your food. If this is not effective, take 300 mg. salt tablets (available over the counter at the pharmacy) twice a day. Be more careful on hot days when you sweat more and collect more leg fluid (edema) and this decreases fluid volume and blood pressure drops. Consult your physician if you have any heart difficulties.

- Exercise your feet and legs before rising from a bed or chair.

- Try sitting with your legs crossed or putting one foot up on a stool or chair.

- Change position slowly. After standing up, support yourself by holding onto someone or something. Cross your legs at or above the knees and squeeze the thigh and/or leg muscles together. This helps the blood to flow upwards ("The cocktail party stance").

- Alcohol dilates blood vessels and lowers blood pressure and may have to be stopped until blood pressure is controlled with some of the other measures outlined above.

- Other drug treatments for postural hypotension may include: reducing or stopping some drugs for Parkinson's. The drugs most likely to aggravate blood pressure drops are: dopamine agonists, selegiline, and anticholinergics (including some antidepressants). Stop any drug slowly. Postural hypotension is a problem as new drugs are added and slow increases can often avoid it.

Therefore if postural hypotension is a significant problem, the following will almost surely help:

- Review all drugs. The first treatment should be to try and remove any medications that are increasing the problem and could be stopped without a major loss of function. **Be especially careful when withdrawing drugs for hypertension as very high blood pressure lying may occur**. Blood pressure must be checked lying and standing.

- Increase salt and caffeine.

- Reduce alcohol.

- Be careful after meals, showers and in hot weather.

- Elevate the head of the bed.

- Use drug therapy to improve control of blood pressure.

- Note the use of drinking water (see tip five previous).

- Check for anemia.

The Digestive System

Patients with Parkinson's may develop very bothersome symptoms and problems involving a number of functions of the gastrointestinal system. **It has been shown that Lewy bodies, which are the marker of the Parkinson's process, are seen in neuronal cells of the digestive system**. Some symptoms are a nuisance, others are very serious and cause major problems which require careful attention. **Difficulty in swallowing is probably the most serious because of poor nutrition and the risk of food aspiration into the lungs. Impaired stomach emptying results in poor medication absorption and can cause motor fluctuations.**

The common gastrointestinal problems include: **drooling, dry mouth, dental care problems, loss of smell and taste, swallowing difficulty, impaired gastric emptying, drug related nausea and vomiting, constipation, weight loss, nutrition and the low protein diet**. These will all be discussed in the next sections.

These are significant symptoms and problems for any person with or without Parkinson's. If the symptom is of sudden onset, and not responding to treatment, then more extensive investigations to rule out other causes may be indicated. **The occurrence and severity of these problems is usually related to the duration and severity of the disability itself rather than treatment and this is especially true for constipation**. Therefore management of these symptoms usually should not include a decrease in antiparkinson medication but rather a treatment which enhances this therapy **and all of these symptoms may be improved.**

Drooling

Difficulty and **slowness in swallowing along** with the **lowered head position** and the tendency to keep the **mouth open** causes excessive pooling of saliva. **This leads to drooling** which is usually first a problem at night. **Production of saliva in parkinsonians is normal**. The treatment of severe drooling is not completely satisfactory. Some of the measures outlined below will help and there is optimism for the future as new drugs are used that reduce saliva production without causing side effects.

Tips for Drooling

• Concentrate on holding the head up, deliberately closing the mouth and swallowing.

• Try to swallow a little more often instead of letting the saliva pool in your mouth.

• Drug changes may help. Drugs with anticholinergic properties may give some relief. But confusion must be watched for. Ditropan (see section on Bladder) causes dry mouth and might help as it has a low risk of confusion).

• Remind yourself to swallow by sucking a mint or chewing gum.

• Atropine has been effective in preventing drooling. The method involves wetting a Q-tip and adding one drop of atropine eye drops (1%) to it. Rub and rotate the Q-tip on one side of the mouth underneath the tongue and then repeat for the other side. Apply one to two times daily. This method has been less helpful than hoped for but worth a try.

• Propantheline (15-45 mg/day), a peripherally acting anticholinergic may help. Side effects include, dilated pupils (watch in glaucoma), urine retention, constipation, fast heart rate, drowsiness, insomnia, and decreased taste. A drug used for ulcers (Pirenzepine) which blocks saliva over production caused by Clozapine has been used in Germany with good results and few side effects. It is possible that it may be helpful in Parkinson's.

- Chewing on and keeping a clove (regular kitchen variety) in the mouth for several hours has been reported to significantly reduce drooling in some patients.

- Preliminary studies with botulinum toxin injections into the glands that produce saliva have shown benefit.

Dry Mouth and Mouth Care Advice

Dry mouth is a common side effect of anticholinergics like Artane or Cogentin and tricyclic antidepressants and also Ditropan used for urinary frequency. The dryness comes from a reduced flow of saliva and is often most noticeable when beginning new drug therapy. It tends to become less apparent as therapy continues. Dry mouth may also be a result of breathing with the mouth open. Some patients just have dry mouth and it is not related to medication.

Tips for Dry Mouth and Mouth Care

- Suck on a mint or sour candy.

- Chew gum.

- Use a mouth spray.

- The tongue may become stuck to the roof of the mouth. If this occurs use a straw and suck up water to lubricate the mouth and then repeat.

- Drink more fluids.

- Try an oral rinse, which can act as a saliva substitute. These rinses can be obtained from a pharmacist.

- Sip water frequently or melt ice in your mouth.

- Reduce caffeine intake.

- Use a humidifier in the room where you sleep.

- If your teeth are sensitive, ask your dentist about topical fluoride gel.

- Use proper oral hygiene techniques such as brushing teeth and flossing regularly. An electric toothbrush can be effective for individuals with less muscle control.

- For dry lips, apply a lubricant such as hydrous lanolin or K-Y Jelly, but not a petroleum based product, as it makes the lips dryer.

- Avoid alcohol and tobacco, as they tend to dry out the mouth. Many mouthwashes also contain large amounts of alcohol and should be avoided.

- A recent study found that an oral drug called pilocarpine improved salvia production, however most patients manage quite well with the above suggestions.

Dental Care

Patients who have troublesome tremor or are slow in their everyday activities may neglect their teeth. Good dental hygiene is important to your health. Poor dental care causes infection, discomfort and difficulty in eating. **Establish a good relationship with a dentist and make regular visits.**

Tips for Dental Care

- Visit your dentist every six months. If tremor or poor mobility are problems, you could be referred to a dentist who specializes in treating patients with medical problems. Many hospitals have dental clinics.

- Lengthen or thicken the toothbrush handle with an assistive device.

- Use an electric toothbrush.

- Clean dentures with a nailbrush attached to the sink with suction cups. These can be purchased and will allow denture cleaning with one hand.

- The caregiver should monitor and assist with dental care if necessary.

Loss of Smell and Taste

Recently, it has been discovered that patients with Parkinson's and progressive supranuclear palsy differ significantly in their ability to smell. This finding may prove to be an effective method of distinguishing earlier which illness an individual may have. It was found that patients with Parkinson's have a decreased sense of smell due to damage of the dopamine cells in the olfactory (smell) system. **The senses of taste and smell are intimately interconnected and a loss in the capacity to smell may contribute to weight loss**. Patients may eat less because of decreased enjoyment of food. Meals may be more palatable if extra attention is given to both the texture and eye appeal of food. Increased use of spices, herbs and other flavouring agents can also help to make up for decreased sensitivity to taste.

Swallowing Difficulty

Swallowing difficulties (dysphagia) of some degree may occur in up to 40% of Parkinson's patients. If severe, it may result in impaired nutrition and chest infections from food getting into the lungs. It is usually **more severe with solids than liquids**. Aging itself also causes a progressive slowing of these functions. Both difficulties in moving the food around inside the mouth and passage of food to the back of the throat may be noted because of a reduction in tongue movement. Some people may find it difficult to initiate the swallow promptly. Others may find that food or pills stick in the sides of the throat after the swallow is completed and coughing results. This will contribute to poor medication effect. This may be due to a weakness in the muscles of the throat, which would normally act to push the food through the throat, and into the esophagus or food channel. **When swallowing impairment is significant, up to 30% of patients will also have associated respiratory symptoms including cough, choking, and shortness of breath at night. Your clinic treatment team may further assess your degree of swallowing difficulty** by having you swallow three ounces of water. Coughing and a wet hoarse voice in the minute after swallowing indicate a risk for lung problems (aspiration). This test will predict about 80% of risk for aspiration and a positive test is an indication for more studies. **This degree of difficulty is uncommon and for most patients swallowing difficulties are only a nuisance that can be controlled**. Patients with progressive supranuclear palsy may have more severe problems.

Problems swallowing have social implications, patients feel uncomfortable eating out and the pleasure of eating is reduced. It has been noted that patients frequently do not complain of dysphagia unless asked. If you have this symptom report it.

The most important precautions are: to eat with the chin tucked down and having the proper food texture. Some patients only have swallowing difficulty when they are in an "off" spell; this is important to establish as improving motor fluctuations may significantly improve swallowing. If dysphagia is severe it may be best to try eating only when you have a good medication effect.

There have been reports of complete blockage of the esophagus in patients who have swallowing difficulty and take psyllium for constipation. Compounds that have this are Metamucil and Perdiem. The symptoms are: cannot swallow; much saliva; choking and chest discomfort. This requires emergency treatment in hospital and the mass of granules must be removed.

You will find eating easier, more enjoyable and safer by following the suggestions below.

Tips for Swallowing Difficulty

- Since eating takes longer, try four to six small meals a day instead of three larger ones.

- Cut food into small pieces to make chewing easier.

- Remember to take your time and chew slowly and thoroughly. Do not rush your meals and be careful talking with your mouth full and trying to swallow at the same time.

- Take a sip of liquid after each swallow of solid food.

- Eat soft foods such as chicken, ground meat, stew, thick soup, or meat loaf. Avoid hot dogs and sausages.

- If fluids are difficult to swallow, increase fluid intake by eating jello, sherbet or suck on ice chips or popsicles. There are also food thickeners which can be added to liquids to thicken them slightly therefore making them easier to handle (food starch and for cold drinks = gelatin).

- Use plate warmers so food does not get cold. Food that is at room temperature may not give the sensors in the mouth much stimulation. It is recommended that food be somewhat colder or warmer than room temperature, although be careful not to go too cold or hot.

- Be sure dentures fit properly. It is very difficult to eat (as well as talk), if dentures are not secure.

- To take small sips of liquid. Try a straw.

- Take small sips from a full glass. This allows your head to be in a better position when swallowing, instead of tilting the head far back to get the last drops.

- Foods that do not need to be chewed, such as yogurt and applesauce may be placed further back on the tongue to reduce the problem of moving the food backwards with the tongue.

- When consuming more solid foods, swallow two or more times before taking more.

- For taking medication: try chewing a banana or using warm applesauce or some other pureed fruit and add the pills. This allows the pills to slide down more easily.

- Drug changes help little and anticholinergics may worsen swallowing however as noted above if swallowing is worse with "off" spells then improving them will help. Amantadine helps stroke patients to swallow and prevents pneumonia. This might be a consideration for Parkinson's patients.

- Special x-rays (supervised barium swallow) can be taken to indicate the specific problem with your swallowing. If necessary, this will be recommended by your doctor or speech pathologist.

- Put no more than a half of one teaspoon in your mouth at one time.

- Completely empty your mouth by swallowing several times, before adding more food or liquid.

- Do not mix liquids and solids in your mouth.

- To prevent food or liquid from going down the wrong way, **lower your chin towards your chest and then swallow**. This is most important. Keep your head down and swallow again. Always sit up to eat. Throwing the head back to swallow may propel food or pills into the airway.

- If your voice sounds wet after swallowing, swallow again.

- Intensive voice training has improved swallowing (see section on Speech).

- There are some throat operations done for severe swallowing difficulty (cricopharyngeal myotomy). This is an option only after extensive discussion with an ear, nose and throat specialist or chest surgeon. It is major surgery.

- A feeding tube may be permanently placed in the stomach or upper small bowel through a small abdominal incision. Only a few patients require this.

- Patients who have swallowing difficulty should not use psyllium containing compounds for constipation as discussed in the introduction above.

- Family members of patients having swallowing problems should learn the Heimlich maneuver to clear an obstruction from the airway. As well, patients may want to learn how to perform the Heimlich maneuver on themself. If a patient finds themself choking, they should make a fist and place the thumb side of that fist against the abdomen, just above the navel. The other hand should then grasp the fist and press inwards and upwards with quick sharp thrusts. Another method to use if choking is to press your abdomen forcefully against the back of a chair, table, sink or hand railing. Repeat this move until the object has been removed. The formal Heimlich maneuver can be learned through various groups that give first aid and emergency management courses.

- Home suction devices are available for patients who have intermittent severe excess saliva and choking episodes.

Tips For Food Preparation to Ease Swallowing

- There are a number of food ideas that will greatly reduce the risk of both choking and getting food into the lungs. **Foods that increase risk include sticky foods**: peanut butter, fresh white bread, dry mashed potatoes, bagels, caramel, sticky buns, thick fudge or butterscotch sauce. **Also foods with small pits**: olives, citrus fruits with seeds, cherries, or grapes. **Foods of two or more consistencies**: citrus fruits, yogurt with fruit, or soups containing vegetables and/or macaroni. **Foods with stringy fibers**: celery, spinach, fennel or asparagus. **Foods that do not easily form a proper mass** (bolus) to swallow: raw fruits, thin pureed fruits, coconut, raisins, corn, peas, mixed vegetables, nuts, seeds, plain ground meats, dry crackers and bread, plain rice, popcorn, bran (grape nut) and shredded wheat cereals.

• To moisten foods: use gravy, sauces, butter or cream.

• To change consistency: chop and chew, mince, or puree with liquid to make an applesauce like consistency.

Impaired Gastric Emptying

Stomach emptying is slow in Parkinson's. It is variable and may be seen early in some patients even before treatment and others have very little. **The symptoms are: a sensation of fullness, feeling satisfied almost immediately after eating, nausea, bloating, and discomfort after meals**. Occasionally there may be vomiting. This problem may also reduce the effect of medication, as drugs must get out of the stomach into the small intestine to be absorbed. Levodopa doses may just sit in the stomach and there may be a very slow (up to 2 hours) or no effect. Patients who have motor fluctuations have much more impaired stomach emptying and this may be the major cause in some patients. **This may be significantly helped by drugs which promote stomach emptying such as domperidone or cisapride**. Some patients with motor fluctuations have had improvement in Parkinson's medication effect with the use of cisapride, which has given less episodes of non-responsiveness to drugs and a shorter time to onset of effect. **Cisapride** increases acetylcholine (cholinergic) function in the stomach neuronal system and this improves stomach emptying and also colonic contraction (improves constipation). Cisapride should not be used if cardiac rhythm is not normal, if there is liver or kidney abnormality and with some antibiotics and antifungal drugs. **Domperidone** improves stomach emptying, bloating and heartburn but not constipation. In some patients, selegiline or Sinemet may cause chronic nausea, and bloating is a rare side effect of bromocriptine therapy. Tricyclic antidepressants may occasionally cause chronic nausea.

Tips to Improve Gastric Emptying and Medication Effect

- Take levodopa on an empty stomach at least 30 minutes before food. If possible, after the dose, move around and avoid lying down.

- Chew or crush Sinemet. Use lots of water to either drink or mix it in. Carbonated drinks may help.

- Much more soluble forms of levodopa are being developed (levodopa ethylester).

- Avoid anticholinergic drugs, they slow gastric emptying.

- Take cisapride or domperidone (really helps nausea) to improve stomach emptying. May just need to take before doses of levodopa that usually fail.

- It may be helpful to take a larger dose at the times you know the onset of effect is always slow or nil (most common with afternoon doses).

- Try levodopa in liquid form. This method should be set up for you by your treatment team. It basically involves taking a 12 to 14 hour total amount of levodopa, mixing it in water and taking a specific amount every hour over the time for example between 7am and 7pm. You then take regular or slow release Sinemet before bed and during the night. This is only done with levodopa not the other drugs. Mixed in the morning and kept cool (not necessary if out of the home) it is stable in solution. Adding vitamin C is not necessary. This method is worth a try, some patients find it cumbersome.

- A tube directly into the small bowel is rarely needed for impaired stomach emptying.

Drug Related Nausea and Vomiting

Nausea and vomiting may occur because of the drug treatment of Parkinson's. Levodopa by itself induces vomiting but when combined with carbidopa or benserazide, vomiting and nausea decrease markedly and are usually transient. Only about 10% of patients have gastric upset (usually nausea) if Sinemet 100/25 is used to start treatment. If the patient has been on medication for a long time and still has poor appetite and some nausea, the doctor should consider a preparation with more carbidopa, for example Sinemet 100/25 instead of 100/10. If stomach symptoms develop during treatment; tests may be indicated to rule out causes not related to Parkinson's. Remember; impaired gastric emptying can also cause this.

Tips for Nausea and Vomiting

- Take levodopa or dopamine agonist drugs on a full stomach. Later on you may be able to take them on an empty stomach and patients with motor fluctuations may note a better drug effect without food.

- If medication is taken other than at mealtimes, then take with a light snack or some milk.

- Try more carbidopa if on Sinemet. For example instead of Sinemet 100/10, use 100/25.

- Try levodopa-benserazide capsules (Prolopa or Madopar).

- Your doctor may prescribe domperidone (10-20 mg three times daily one hour before eating). Domperidone does not cause drug-induced parkinsonism because it blocks dopamine receptors only in the brain stem vomiting centre and does not gain access to basal ganglia dopamine receptors. It may be used in the first months of levodopa or dopamine agonist therapy. It also improves stomach emptying. Mild drowsiness occasionally occurs

- Review all other drugs with your doctor, for example; drugs for arthritis frequently cause stomach upset.

- Selegiline may cause chronic nausea and tricyclic antidepressants are an uncommon cause.

Constipation

This affects about 50% of Parkinson's patients and causes much distress. It may also cause gas pain, abdominal distension, hemorrhoids and oozing of liquid stool. **It is the most common gastrointestinal symptom of Parkinson's. Contributing factors include**: involvement of the nerve supply of the colon by the Parkinson's process resulting in slow transit time through the colon; insufficient intake of fluid and bulk; general weakness and loss of strength to push; and sometimes ignoring the urge.

Patients must remember that it is normal not to have a bowel movement everyday. Constipation is often defined as less than three bowel movements per week. **With careful management, almost all patients obtain excellent control of this bothersome component of the illness**. You will have to develop your own individual bowel management program and once established, stick to it and avoid recurring bouts of more severe constipation. **A high fibre diet, with or without laxatives, is almost always effective.**

There may also be abnormalities related to the rectum and anus. The problem of bowel outlet difficulty has only been recognized recently and has been referred to as **pelvic floor muscle dystonia**. Instead of the normal relaxation of these muscles during a bowel movement, they go into spasm. Laxatives will not help this. Cisapride (5mg twice daily) has proven to be a useful drug for motor disorders of the gut. It promotes release of acetylcholine and has no central effects and therefore does not lead to confusion. **Cisapride may promote normalization of these anorectal relaxation reflexes and has helped severe constipation**

Constipation may rarely be very severe and lead to obstruction. Enemas with bethanecol have been reported to help if other measures fail. The sudden onset of acute abdominal pain in a patient with severe chronic constipation suggests a twisted bowel (sigmoid volvulus) which requires emergency surgery.

If you have constipation, report it, help is available.

Factors Contributing to Constipation

- Lack of daily exercise

- Not enough bulk and fibre in the diet

- Decreased muscle power generally

- Limited fluid intake

- Depression

- Medication including:

    - some antiparkinsonian drugs, for example those with anticholinergic effect (stop slowly)

    - antacids, for example Amphojel, Maalox

    - diuretics

    - antiarthritic agents such as non-steroidals which may also cause bleeding

    - pain medications containing codeine

Tips for Constipation

It is best to try natural means. You are advised to:

- Eat meals at regular times.

- Increase bulk and high fibre in diet. Choose:

    - whole grain breads and cereals

    - 100% whole wheat bread, oatmeal, Red River cereal, Shreddies, Bran and shredded wheat

- rice and pasta

  - fruits - raw or with skins, dried fruits (if you have trouble swallowing, try a blender). Bananas worsen constipation and should not be used.

  - leafy vegetables - lettuce, broccoli, celery

  - bran may be sprinkled over cereal, added to baked goods (muffins), meatloaf or casseroles.

  - lentils, split peas and barley

- Too much fiber can cause bloating.

- Establish regular bowel habits. Preferably 30 minutes after a meal at the same time each day. Recall your normal pattern and try to return to it.

- Increase your fluid intake to 4-8 glasses daily. This is most important

  - Preferably water - keep water near your chair and heating it may improve the enjoyment. Do not count tea and coffee. Use fruit juices especially prune, plum, peach and pear

- Participate in regular exercise such as a 10-minute daily walk.

- Try senna tea or prune juice.

- Hot beverages, including hot water have a laxative effect and are best taken in the morning.

- If these methods are not effective, it may be necessary to use laxatives. There are many different types available:

- Bulk Laxatives: increase the stool bulk and promote easier movement of the bowels, for example Fibyrax or Metamucil - one or more teaspoons twice daily in a large glass of water. Do not use them if you have difficulty swallowing (see section on Swallowing). The use of bulking agents must be accompanied by a high liquid intake (at least 8 glasses per day) or it may actually worsen constipation. It should be noted that abuse of laxatives could cause diarrhea.

- Stool Softeners: promote softer and more regular bowel movements, for example Docusate (Colace) - one capsule once or twice daily. The onset of effect is delayed and you should continue all the other above measures.

- Milk of magnesia (two tablespoons) if bulk and softeners do not work.

- Irritant laxatives: Ex-Lax, Feen-a-Mint, Correctal, Dulcolax are best avoided. Use once per week at most. Chronic use will disrupt normal bowel contractions and the bowel becomes lazy. Long term use of mineral oil can interfer with absorption of vitamins minerals and drugs.

- Lactulose solution (15 to 60 cc daily) may benefit some patients.

- Enemas may be useful once per week if necessary.

- The following recipe for fruit spread may help. The ingredients are 2/3 cup of raisins, 10 dates, 10 prunes,

1/4 cup of molasses, and 1/2 cup of natural bran. Soak the prunes in water overnight. Put the juice aside. Combine the raisins, dates, prunes, and juice of the prunes together in a blender. Mix well. Add molasses and bran. Transfer mixture to a casserole. Bring to a boil then reduce heat and let simmer 10 minutes. Refrigerate and serve cold. Use two tablespoons one to three times daily at mealtime on a muffin, cereal or with other food or hot water. Another simple routine is to use prunes daily. Eat three to four per day and soak a few days supply overnight in the fridge in water.

Note: It may be necessary to use a combination of all of the above including both bulk laxatives and a stool softener daily. Patients can easily manage this program. When purchasing laxatives or stool softeners over the counter, be sure to discuss the different options with the pharmacist. If constipation continues, your personal physician should be consulted. Occasionally patients require other drugs or regular enemas. **A good simple starting plan is to: increase fluid and use bran and prunes daily.**

Weight Loss, Nutrition and the Low Protein Diet

There is no specific diet for most patients with Parkinson's. However a good diet with three balanced meals per day with a recommended (five to one) balance of carbohydrate and protein, is important. **Parkinson's patients are four times more likely to lose ten or more pounds than other people of the same age.**

Some patients may slowly lose weight. Other causes should be excluded but Parkinson's itself can, and usually is, a factor.

Metabolism is increased in Parkinson's and those patients with the most severe increased tone and involuntary movements have the highest energy expenditure. It is suspected that there also is a defect in energy production. **In addition, caloric intake may be reduced due to**: slowness in eating; difficulty in cutting, chewing, and swallowing food; reduced absorption from the gut; failure to complete meals in the required time; difficulty handling food items; and poor dental health or poor fitting dentures which make chewing difficult. Any infection will promote rapid weight loss. Depression, anxiety and memory loss (see section on Memory Disorders) may be significant factors and this should be carefully assessed.

Weight loss can be a significant problem for some more advanced Parkinson's patients. Even though caloric intake and appetite remain stable, weight still decreases. Calories must be increased to maintain a consistent weight. There are supplements available such as Ensure and Sustacal but these are expensive and milkshakes or instant breakfast may be just as beneficial. A referral to a dietician for a review of your diet will be helpful. The dietician will be able to suggest foods of high caloric density.

Patient's who have unilateral pallidotomy or bilateral subthalamic nucleus stimulation gain weight after the procedure. The reasons may be: decreased dyskinesias, better mobility and access to food, ease in eating and reduced anxiety and depression.

Tips to Increase Weight

• Serve six small meals a day instead of three larger ones. This reduces the time and effort required eating.

- Make use of assistive devices to help handle the food (see section on Assistive Devices and Techniques).

- Request a referral to a speech and swallowing pathologist to determine the cause of the swallowing problem. They will also give you advice to make swallowing easier (see section on Swallowing Difficulty).

- Pay extra attention to dental care. More frequent dental visits may be necessary (see section on Dental Care). Be sure dentures fit properly.

- Consult a dietitian regarding foods with a high caloric content.

- Pay attention to food preparation.

- Carefully review if depression or anxiety are factors.

- If preparation is a problem - use the Meals on Wheels service.

- Weight loss that is sudden in onset and progresses quickly deserves more review especially if there are other symptoms.

Excess carbohydrate intake may aggravate dyskinesias. The mechanism is as follows: excess carbohydrate causes more insulin release, which reduces large neutral amino acids and allows more dopamine in the brain. The patient and family observing any change after a good sweet fix can easily settle this. **Candy and other goodies should be a great enjoyment and source of calories for patients and their use is encouraged**. There is no evidence that this has any bad effect on Parkinson's.

Excess protein can make motor fluctuations worse as large neutral amino acids may block both the absorption of levodopa from the intestine and its entry into the brain. This observation has led to the use of a low protein diet for patients with motor fluctuations. **The concept is: that protein is restricted at breakfast and lunch and the protein for the day is taken at supper**. Parkinson patients should be aware that they might be slower after a very high protein meal.

Before trying this, consult your neurologist or nurse coordinator and then a dietician or nutritionist. Remember: **the protein adjustments are only helpful in patients with motor fluctuations** and for most patients only a regular balanced diet is needed. The protein theory is not completely accepted. Some believe that if levodopa gets out of the stomach, then it is absorbed quickly and is effective with no relation to protein. The low protein diet has helped some patients. **Few patients use it long term and there are some disadvantages**. Protein intake may be inadequate; weight loss may result; transient confusion and depression have been noted; and the patient must face the predictable and perhaps more severe slowness that follows the high protein evening meal. Carefully managed however, it may be a useful treatment option for healthy, highly motivated patients with excellent nutritional status. If it is going to work then it is obvious in the first week. A much easier approach is to take levodopa on an empty stomach one hour before or after meals. Most patients can tolerate this.

Vitamin B6, if taken in large quantities can be a problem for patients using plain levodopa (not Sinemet, Prolopa or Madopar). Patients taking B6 should not eliminate it totally as it plays an important role in your diet. Pyridoxine (B6) can stimulate the enzyme which converts levodopa to dopamine.

Therefore by the time the levodopa reaches the brain it is in the dopamine form. Dopamine cannot cross the blood-brain barrier so the original levodopa has become ineffective in combating parkinsonism symptoms. **Very few patients are on plain levodopa and therefore pyridoxine is not an issue for most Parkinson's patients.**

Fractures, Osteoporosis and Prevention

Patients with Parkinson's have a higher incidence of bone thinning (osteoporosis) than the general population of the same age. Also patients with more loss of mobility have greater bone loss. Fractures, and especially hip fractures, are common in Parkinson's patients because of their increased tendency to fall. Every attempt should be made to decrease this. **Osteoporosis is a major contributing factor to the fracture tendency and a concerted effort should be made to prevent, diagnose and treat osteoporosis.** This is especially important for females and should be part of the treatment plan. Osteoporosis does occur in males and is felt to be inadequately appreciated or treated. Inactivity increases osteoporosis and this again **underlines the importance of being active and following an exercise program** (especially weight bearing, walking, dancing). Swimming is also excellent for bone building. Calcium supplements and the risks and benefits of estrogen therapy should be discussed with your physician. A new class of estrogen compounds = selective estrogen receptor modulators (SERMs) have been developed and they give bone and heart protection without the breast and uterine cancer risk. Alendronate (Fosamax) has been shown to reduce postmenopausal bone loss and is being used to prevent osteoporosis. This is an excellent drug. **These therapies clearly reduce bone loss and the fracture risk**. Established osteoporosis (especially spinal) will be helped with vitamin D, calcium, estrogen, etidronate (Didrocal) and Alendronate. **Osteoporosis is diagnosed by having a bone mineral density test**. This is easy to do and widely available and can follow the response to treatment. The treatment of osteoporosis is changing and complex and you should have a treatment plan made by an endocrinologist or internist.

Facts About Osteoporosis

- Osteoporosis risk is increased in: females, increased age, ovarian removal, chronic oral cortisone use, early menopause, insufficient dietary calcium and excess alcohol and tobacco use.

- A bone mineral density test can predict the fracture risk and follow treatment.

- A woman age 50 has a 15% chance of a hip fracture in her remaining lifetime.

- Bone density is decreased in Parkinson's (because of off periods and bradykinesia) and fracture risk is higher in both males and females.

- In addition to daily weight bearing exercise, calcium supplementation slows bone loss. The best sources are milk, cheese and yogurt. Two cups of milk daily provides 600 mg. of calcium plus Vitamin D, which helps absorb calcium. Extra strength Tums provide 300 mg. of calcium in each tablet and patients (especially with more disability and less sunlight) often should be on vitamin D 1000 units a day.

• Estrogen therapy after menopause clearly reduces osteoporosis. Bone loss is slower in the early postmenopausal years and a life long treatment plan should be developed using all of the treatments outlined in varying combination. The important point here is that osteoporosis in late life, when falls are more frequent should and can be prevented.

Therefore all Parkinson's patients should work to prevent osteoporosis. Spine and limb fractures are very painful and disabling and are associated with increased mortality.

Speech (Dysarthria)

Parkinson's patients commonly experience problems with both speech and voice. However, not everyone will have difficulty and should they develop problems, they may be of varying types and degree. The voice may become very weak so it is difficult to be heard. Sometimes the voice may be strong enough at the beginning of a sentence but fade as the sentence progresses. **Recent studies have given better understanding of the problem. Detailed electrical testing has shown reduced activity in the muscles of the larynx, face and jaw. All of these contribute to the low voice and in addition reduced facial expression makes it more difficult for the listener**. Direct observation of the larynx during speech shows reduced movement and tremor that does not improve with levodopa but speech may be louder after levodopa probably from better function of the face, lips, and chest. Remember speech is produced by air coming out of the lungs and crossing the vocal cords in the larynx (voice box). The larynx makes complex movements, which set the air into vibration and the lips, tongue and cheeks then shape it into speech. Breathing problems will reduce volume.

Levodopa therapy may improve low volume speech initially. The sound of the voice may be a monotone, lacking expression or intonation. Speech may lack clarity and precision due to difficulty in articulating clearly. The rate of speaking may be affected, that is, phrase rushes may occur and it becomes very difficult to slow the speech down. Some patients find they repeat sounds or words almost as though they are stuttering. Difficulty in initiation of speech can occur as well as inappropriate silences. Although many patients manage quite well and do not consider the speech or voice problems to be too disruptive, some will have greater involvement of speech/voice which can significantly compromise their communication needs. The effect of pallidotomy on speech has been assessed (see section on Current Surgical Treatments - Lesioning Procedures).

In addition to the speech and voice problems, some patients may develop word-finding difficulty, which is not necessarily related to intellectual impairment. Writing difficulties may be manifested as micrographia, where the written words become very small and difficult to read.

Intensive voice treatment (the Lee Silverman Voice Treatment - LSVT) focusing on vocal loudness and sensory perception **has given significant voice improvement that was still present at six months**. The program is high effort and very intense involving 16 sessions (4 per week for 4 weeks). Swallowing was also significantly improved.

The following suggestions can help in the management of the above speech or voice problems. Also a formal referral to a speech-language pathologist (speech therapist) will be of benefit.

Tips for Speech

Before beginning to speak:

- *Take time to organize your thoughts and plan what you are going to say.*

- *Swallow before you speak, since there may be a lot of saliva in your mouth, which will make it difficult to speak clearly.*

- *Check that your dentures fit properly. It is very difficult to speak if dentures are loose.*

- *Remember to take a breath before speaking to keep the voice stronger.*

When speaking:

- Try to keep your head upright and look at the person your are talking with. It really does help to be able to see a person's mouth movements.

- Express your ideas in short, concise phrases or sentences.

- Speak clearly. Every word is important. It may help to exaggerate the syllables.

- If the voice is weak, try not to speak in noisy situations. This could be in the car, on the street with traffic noises, at home with the television on or in other situations with a noisy background. Wait until it is quieter.

- Remember to take little catch breaths as you speak and do not try to say too much on one breath. This will help keep the voice strong.

- Use as much inflection in the voice as possible.

- Try to use as much facial expression as you can. Practicing facial exercises in the mirror each day can be helpful (smile, frown, look surprised, etc.).

- To help keep your speech a little more deliberate and paced and avoid rushes in your speech, you may try using a pacing device such as a "pacing board." A speech pathologist can help you with this. Initially try a ruler with clear divisions on it and move your finger along saying one word per division.

- Exercises for the lips, tongue and jaw may help to keep the speech muscles strong. Look into a mirror to see how well you are doing.

- Practice your speech. Read aloud into a tape recorder and then play it back, listening for parts that could be improved.

- If the volume of your voice is extremely weak and it is very difficult to be heard in some situations, you may benefit from a portable voice amplifier. Bell Canada has a voice amplifier that is attached inside the speaker of the telephone. A Speech Pathologist could provide information on the various types of voice amplifiers available. There are new portable battery powered models.

- For those patients whose Parkinson's is advanced there are small communication devices available. These are like small typewriters and the message appears on a screen or on paper printout. Some also have voice outputs.

- An operation to help weak voices involves "adjusting" the vocal cords. However, the results are variable and this procedure is not appropriate for everyone. A Speech Pathologist and Otolaryngologist should be consulted in these cases.

- Read booklets on speech problems and suggested exercises. Various Parkinson's Associations may provide these.

- Discuss referral to Speech Pathology with your doctor or Home Care nurse.

- Clonazepam (0.25-0.5 mg/dose) has helped speech rate and rushes, but not low volume and breathy quality.

- Remember, talk for yourself, and do not let others do it for you.

- Do not shy away from telling others about the way in which Parkinson's has affected your speech. This may make them better listeners and allow them to help you. Educate your friends and family!

- Inquire about some of the intensive speech improvement programs like LSVT. Get the opinion of your speech therapist.

- A light note to end on. Clearly your voice is softer, but those around you have lost hearing and are usually reluctant to admit it. A hearing device might help both of you.

Skin Problems and Care

Parkinson's patients commonly have problems with their skin. These are as follows: oily facial skin, eyelid problems, dry body skin and sweating abnormalities.

Facial Skin

Excessive oil on the skin especially around the scalp and face may occur, resulting in dandruff, scaly skin and eyelid irritation. The oily skin is part of Parkinson's and is more prominent in the central part of the face and the forehead where sebaceous (sweat) glands are more numerous. This is called **seborrheic dermatitis** and is usually easily controllable with proper skin care.

Tips for Facial Skin Care

- Avoid excess moisture on the face. Keep it dry and clean. Limited use of some cosmetics may be beneficial.

- Use water-based (oil free) moisturizing lotions, for example, Lubriderm and water-based make-up.

- Use a mild (drying) soap for washing skin, for example, Dove, Neutrogena, Sunlight or baby soap.

- Use a mild dandruff shampoo like Head and Shoulders for the scalp. Coal tar shampoos (use only twice weekly) are helpful as is topical ketoconazole (Nizoral cream or shampoo).

- Wash the affected facial areas frequently.

- If persistent, see your family physician or a dermatologist. Preparations containing hydrocortisone are sometimes used for the short term and are most helpful.

Eyelids

This is called **blepharitis** and is related to the facial skin problems. Reduced blinking also contributes to the inflammation. If severe this can lead to corneal problems (keratitis).

Tips for Eyelid Care

- Apply artificial tears and warm compresses three or four times daily.

- Steroid cream if more severe.

- Eye patches at bedtime if blinking is severely impaired. This is to avoid corneal abrasions during sleep.

Dry Body Skin

Parkinson's seems to create an oily face and hair yet the rest of the body is very dry (Xerosis). Therefore something applicable to the face and hair may not be recommended for the body. Immobility, malnutrition, excess perspiration, or incontinence can cause skin breakdown.

Tips for Body Skin Care

- Take fewer showers (every second day), so the skin will not become too dry.

- Apply perfume-free moisturizing creams like gloxal base, dermabase or petroleum jelly (Vaseline).

- Keep active, including exercise.

- Keep a normal weight. To keep healthy skin a proper balanced diet needs to be maintained.

- If you are restricted to bed or confined to a wheelchair, reposition yourself at least every two hours to avoid pressure on your skin. Sheepskin pads or air cushions will help to prevent bedsores. These are available at health supply stores.

Sweating Abnormalities

Excessive sweating and temperature control problems are part of Parkinson's. **The cause is felt to be Parkinson's involvement of the central (hypothalamus) and peripheral nervous system parts that control these functions**. Abnormal sensations of heat or cold, impaired sweating, and low body temperature (hypothermia) may occur. Some patients have excess sweating of the face and neck with increased environmental temperature and this is related to impaired heat loss control. It may be made worse by exertion, fever or anxiety. Most sweating problems occur in patients with more severe disability. Levodopa therapy for the treatment of parkinsonism tends to initially improve excessive sweating. Later, **bouts of severe sweating are more usually related to periods of slowness but may also occur during "on" periods with dyskinesias**. The "off" period sweating will often be improved with measures to reduce motor fluctuations such as dopamine agonists. The sweating that occurs with "on" periods is usually not as bad and will respond to medication reduction but often with an increase in slow time. These patients with peak dose sweating are more likely to be helped with beta-blocker drugs (like propranolol) than are those with "off" sweating. Severe fever and sweating may develop after sudden stopping of levodopa (malignant hyperthermia). This takes several days to develop and may be extremely serious and therefore, if possible, levodopa should always be withdrawn slowly.

Parkinson's does not cause all excess sweating and other causes should ruled out. High doses of alcohol or aspirin; overactive thyroid; infections; menopause; and some tumors are other possible causes. The question of whether levodopa causes melanoma or the recurrence of melanoma was raised early in its use. Long-term experience indicates that **levodopa is not involved in the growth or recurrence of melanoma** and that it can be used safely in Parkinson's patients who have had melanoma. Other studies have shown that levodopa has an antitumor effect on melanoma.

Tips for Sweating

- Increase fluid intake, especially in warm weather.

- Keep a facecloth or towel handy.

- Bring an extra set of clothing if sweating is severe and you are going out.

- Dress by the weather report in the winter. You may feel warm and not dress for cold weather.

- Athletic types of clothing (tracksuit or t-shirt) are useful, as they absorb the sweat.

- Some patients have severe episodic sweats. As noted above, the sweating spells must be timed to medication effect to determine the proper treatment. Watch for blood pressure drop with propranolol or dopamine agonist addition.

- Have a careful general review to rule out causes not related to Parkinson's.

Foot Pain and Foot Care

Foot pain and deformities are common in older patients generally, and are often a bothersome problem for patients with

Parkinson's. Some of the problems may be treatment related. Leg pain, foot pain and flexing or extending of the toes may occur because of rigidity or prolonged levodopa treatment resulting in **dystonia. Foot cramps** may cause the muscles of the foot to go into spasm, which positions the toes into a claw-like form. **Some of these foot problems may respond to medication adjustments** (see sections on Dyskinesias, Dystonia, and Pain).

Levodopa-induced dyskinesias may cause abnormal foot and ankle movements when walking which may contribute to imbalance and to the beginning of more persistent foot pain. Various foot and toe deformities occur in patients without Parkinson's. Many are caused by osteoarthritis. In addition patients may have arch problems, deviated or flexed toes, and corns and calluses. Foot pain may also be present only on walking.

Ankle pain is less common, it may be arthritic in origin or related to foot problems. Referral to a rheumatologist is often needed to develop a treatment plan.

Tips for Foot Care

- Wash feet once a day in warm water but not for an extended period of time, as it will dry the foot.

- Massage the feet regularly with a skin cream. Massage in an upward direction from the toes towards the ankle. Avoid massaging if the patient has poor circulation or skin infection.

- Wear footwear that is supportive to the feet, such as lace-up shoes with a low to medium heel. Avoid wearing slippers, as they offer little support. Do not wear restrictive footwear as pressure is caused, resulting in hard skin, bunions and corns. Poor footwear is the most common cause of foot problems.

- Wear hosiery that is large enough to allow movement in the toes.

- If cramping foot pain persists, consult your physician, as medication adjustments may be necessary and will give good relief.

- Cut toenails, once per month, straight across, using clippers. This prevents ingrown toenails.

- If general foot care is difficult for you, then visit a chiropodist or foot clinic. There are many foot clinics available in the community.

- An orthopedic surgeon or rheumatologist with a particular interest in foot problems could be consulted.

Pain and Sensory Symptoms

Fluctuating pain and sensory symptoms are common and affect up to 50% of patients with Parkinson's. The symptoms are variable and inconsistent, taking the form of cramping, numbness, burning, coldness or deep aching. It is usually more in the legs than arms, rarely in the face or neck and worse on the body side most involved with Parkinson's. Pain is more proximal, numbness more in the fingers or toes. The origin of these symptoms is not clear, **they are more in the "off" state and often associated with dystonia**. Abdominal pain may occur. Pain is often associated with clinical motor fluctuations and is much more common if the patient is depressed. It seems to be less frequent and severe when experiencing an "on" period. Dystonia can cause painful spasms, usually in the foot and leg, but may be present in the neck, jaw, trunk, arm or hand. Neck or low back pain may be related to muscle rigidity, arthritis or disc disease. **Antiparkinsonian medication adjustments often decrease the pain and the aim is to decrease slow time**. In a few patients, pain can become quite severe. In these cases, measures to provide more continuous dopamine stimulation (pump, duodenal infusions or slow release levodopa preparations) may alleviate the pain. Lithium has also been useful in dystonic "off" period pain (see sections on Daily Mobility Fluctuations and Sleep Problems).

There should be a careful review for other causes. Arthritis may cause painful hip or shoulder bursitis. Diabetes and vascular disease may be considered. The various pains and sensory symptoms may be seen early before Parkinson's is diagnosed and may clear when medication is started. After ruling out these other health problems, heat, massage, increased activity or elevation of the limbs may relieve the discomfort. This should be discussed with your physician.

Low back pain is common generally and Parkinson's patients frequently have it, often as an initial symptom. It should be assessed and treated carefully. Our patients have had excellent relief with both physiotherapy programs and/or lumbar disc surgery. When present early it may clear with drug therapy and later return as the illness worsens.

Headache occurs often in Parkinson's patients. It does not seem to be related to neck stiffness. Antidepressants improve it, levodopa or dopamine agonist therapy do not give consistent benefit.

Internal tremor is a feeling of tremor inside the chest, abdomen, arms and legs and no tremor is seen. It occurs in up to 40% of Parkinson's patients and is more frequent in those with other sensory symptoms such as aching, burning and tingling. It is brief and episodic, more on one side and lasts five to 30 minutes. It is more during slow spells but the response to medication adjustments is not always good. It is better with relaxation walking or changing body position and minor tranquilizers clearly help. It may precede the onset of Parkinson's and is a useful diagnostic factor that may help in screening patients for Parkinson's before the diagnosis is clear.

Tips for Pain

- For morning pain and early morning cramps, levodopa or a dopamine agonist at night may help (see section on Sleep Problems).

- For pain that occurs when slow closer levodopa doses or a dopamine agonist may help.

- For dystonic pain, benefit may be found using a dopamine agonist or lithium.

- A reduction in levodopa may be necessary.

- A regular, gentle exercise program (see section on Exercise), may reduce the pain or discomfort caused by stiff joints and muscles and stooped posture.

- Use specifically designed cushions to relieve neck or back pain. These are available in health supply stores. This should be discussed with a physiotherapist or occupational therapist to aid you in making the right choice.

- Discuss any pain experienced with your physician and a rheumatologist will help with joint or limb pains.

Shoulder Pain

Shoulder joint pain is a frequent problem in Parkinson's. Commonly called "frozen shoulder", it includes pain, a limited range of motion, and stiffness. It occurs because of decreased arm swing and shoulder movement. **Frozen shoulder has been noted before the appearance of the main symptoms of Parkinson's and it affects the body side first affected**. It is seen more in patients with slowness and stiffness rather than tremor and has been noted to clear after thalamotomy. Initiation of antiparkinsonian therapies will often improve this problem. Also range of motion exercises and moving the shoulder with heat (warm shower), will help significantly (see Section on Exercise). Anti-inflammatory drugs such as aspirin or ibuprofen will help. If shoulder pain becomes severe and persistent, a referral to physiotherapy or a rheumatologist is recommended.

Biceps tendonitis may also cause shoulder pain and may result from the forward shoulder posture that some parkinsonians develop. The patient has tenderness of the biceps tendon over the front of the shoulder (see section on Exercise).

The clavicle and shoulder are often injured in falls and very unpleasant chronic shoulder region pain results. This is another good reason to avoid falls (see section on Movement).

Leg Swelling (Edema)

Edema or lower leg swelling is seen often in Parkinson's. If the swelling occurs in both legs, it may be a result of antiparkinsonian drugs especially Symmetrel (amantadine). Dopamine agonists also cause some leg swelling. Also non-steroidal anti-inflammatory drugs cause fluid retention. Edema is often seen if there is a marked weight gain or a decrease in activity, such as that resulting from bradykinesia (slowness). It also may be a sign of kidney or heart failure (which is also usually accompanied by a shortness of breath). **Discuss with your doctor.**

Tips for Leg Swelling

- Reduce salt intake.

- Drug changes. The edema associated with Symmetrel is usually mild and not a reason to stop the drug. Reducing the dose or taking a dose every second day are options.

- Elevate legs when sitting. A footstool, pillows or another low-seated chair are all effective. Lying down with legs elevated 10-20 minutes, 2-3 times a day is most helpful in reducing swelling.

- Avoid tight stockings (knee-highs) or socks. This is not to be confused with support hose that may be recommended by your doctor.

- Make an effort to increase walking but avoid prolonged standing.

Note: **Swelling of one leg with tenderness in the calf or pain on walking suggests phlebitis**. The risk is higher in patients who are more disabled; have had recent major surgery or had a cast on. This is a serious problem because of the risk of blood clots going to the lungs and a doctor should be consulted immediately.

Shortness of Breath

The air volume per deep breath (vital capacity) is reduced in parkinsonian patients. The problem is worse with repetitive attempts in the same way as patients note hand function decreases with repeat use. It is worse with more disability from Parkinson's and also if the patient has fluctuations and dyskinesias. It has been shown that function may improve with medications for Parkinson's (apomorphine used in research study) but in general the benefit of medication has been modest.

In patients with moderate to severe disability, **decreased respiratory function should be considered during surgery or chest infections**. This is a major surgical risk factor and requires careful preoperative evaluation. Your should be assessed by an internist or respirologist and an appropriate test of pulmonary function should be done. Levodopa or dopamine agonists may cause dyskinesias and this may include the diaphragm and produce irregularities of respiration and a sensation of shortness of breath.

It is now being suggested that **respiratory decrease should be addressed early** as it is slowly progressive. Early initiation of an exercise and chest physiotherapy program may give long term functional benefit.

Tips for Shortness of Breath

- Other causes need to be excluded.

- If it is a result of levodopa therapy, it may be improved with more frequent smaller doses (see section on Dyskinesias and Fluctuations) or adding a dopamine agonist and significantly reducing levodopa.

- Chest exercises to improve chest expansion and air exchange may be beneficial. One such exercise is outlined below:

    - Stand straight with feet slightly apart, knees relaxed and arms at sides.

    - Slowly raise straight arms out from your sides to above your head.

    - At the same time, take a long, deep breath to fill your lungs with air.

    - Then slowly lower your straight arms in front of you, curling your back a little at the same time.

    - Slowly blow all the air out of your lungs as you lower your arms.

    - Repeat this exercise three to five times daily.

- Stop exercise if you feel yourself becoming light-headed.

- An active ongoing exercise program will improve respiratory and cardiac function and reduce shortness of breath.

Visual and Eye Problems

Parkinson's does not cause loss of vision or blindness. **Blurred vision and difficulty in reading, dry eyes and double vision** are fairly common complaints of patients whose illness is longstanding. But even patients early in their illness and before treatment may note some visual disturbances. Atypical parkinsonism (especially PSP) is associated with: inability to look down, double vision, blurred vision, reading problems, burning eyes, light sensitivity, slowing of eye opening and closing, and inability to open the eyes at will. Variable double vision may also occur. The most common reason for blurring of vision especially when focussing or attempting to look at something close is related to medication side effects. The most common drugs causing this are ones with anticholinergic effects like trihexyphenidyl, benztropine and tricyclic antidepressants. These drugs block the receptors that regulate the shape of the eye and this plus the lens becoming more rigid with age cause the near vision difficulty and blurring. Caution must also be observed with these drugs in untreated glaucoma as rarely acute attacks are precipitated. **Occasionally patients have double vision and other visual symptoms during "off" spells** and this responds to medication adjustment. Poor adjustment to low light levels, blurred vision, and spatial, colour and pattern discrimination problems are related to retinal and brain dopamine lack and respond to levodopa. The visual complaints that **occur late in Parkinson's are more related to defects in eye-following movements** than to drug therapy. Like muscles in other parts of the body Parkinson's slows eye muscle movements and if this fatigue affects one eye more than the other then double or blurred vision results. The eyes move with a jerky, rachet-like movement, which requires extra effort and causes tiring.

Treatment for these complaints is often unsatisfactory. A thorough eye exam is needed. Prisms (special corrective lenses) may help double vision while cataracts may need surgery. Large print books, magnifying glasses and devices (such as a ruler) may help to focus, stay on the line and shift to the next line. Many of our patients have had wonderful improvement with cataract removal, it is usually done under local anaesthetic. If dyskinesias are a problem this can be managed. Various aids are available to improve vision and you should ask your eye doctor. **It is most important to gain the best vision you can both** for your enjoyment and safety (reduces falls) so raise visual complaints with your treatment team.

Dry eyes are a frequent problem in normal older adults. Tears are normally spread across the eye by blinking. Bradykinesia reduces movements that you normally do unconsciously and this includes blinking. This reduced eye movement contributes to dry eyes. Irritation, scratchiness or burning results. Drugs with anticholinergic effects also cause dry eyes.

Tips for Dry Eyes

- Use a no tear baby shampoo that does not irritate the eyes. The shampoo may also be rubbed into the eyelid to clean the area of crusts.

- Bath the eyes with warm water or a face cloth.

- Use artificial tears that are available at a drugstore without a prescription. Pull down the lower lid and add one to two drops, three or four times daily. There are various types so try several.

- Your doctor may prescribe an ointment or drops.

Driving

The sense of comfort, convenience and freedom of being able to drive your own vehicle is well recognized. However, these mean little against the legal and moral obligations of not putting others at risk. It has been shown that moderately severe Parkinson's patients (tremor or rigidity on both sides, with serious walking problems or falls) are involved in significantly (ten times) more accidents than normal persons of the same age. Parkinson's patients, with this significant level of disability, were shown to: drive slower, have poor lane position and make more mistakes when attention is divided. This results in more rear end collisions and sideswipe accidents. The lower reaction time may increase stopping distance by one third.

Parkinson's patients not only suffer from loss of motor control but also must take many of the drugs mentioned in this book and possibly others as well. Motor fluctuations and medication side effects decrease coordination and increase risk. The overestimation of one's own driving capability is well established, particularly among males. The patient is therefore advised to abide by the assessment of others. If they are uneasy in the vehicle, that is a strong indicator of caution.

Discussion Points:

- **Having Parkinson's does not necessarily mean you are unsafe to drive.**

- Patients with more severe disability (Hoehn and Yahr stage 3) as described above should be careful and most should not drive.

- If the patient or family feel unsafe, then the person should not be driving.

- Reducing risk by driving only in the daytime, in good weather, on low traffic side streets and back roads, is often a good temporary option.

- Some enhanced driver skill courses are offered (for example 55 alive).

- Motor fluctuations and medication side effects decrease coordination and increase risk.

- Taking taxis is not more costly than maintaining a car. Independence can be preserved, and parking problems and risks avoided.

- If the question of driving ability is indefinite, then a repeat driving test or driving skill assessment should be asked for. If you must stop driving, try and accept it, difficult as it is. Your good record and name, your safety and the safety of others is of paramount importance.

Alcohol

Alcohol has been reported to have some beneficial effects on patients with Parkinson's including decreased tremor, improved speech and enhanced sleep. Nevertheless, alcohol is an addictive substance. For example, patients with problems sleeping may find that alcohol promotes sleep. However, it loses its effect and larger doses may be needed. This in turn leads to disruption of nighttime sleep and increases anxiety levels. Chronic, excess alcohol use can lead to memory loss. As well, excess alcohol has the tendency to cause degeneration in the cerebellum, which leads to problems in balance. Because of the risk of damage to the cerebellum, peripheral nerves and memory, Parkinson's patients should carefully avoid alcohol excess. Also common sense suggests that if your balance is already a bit impaired from Parkinson's, be careful about how much you drink and walking after you drink. **Alcohol should never be used to treat a symptom of Parkinson's.**

Alcohol dilates blood vessels and may worsen a postural fall in blood pressure and may have to be at least temporarily avoided until blood pressure can be improved (see section on Postural Hypotension).

All of this sounds very serious. **However, a drink before dinner, some wine with dinner, or a social drink is quite a reasonable approach** to alcohol use and this is the advice we give our patients. We have rarely seen Parkinson's patients using alcohol to excess.

There have been reports of transient, alcohol withdrawal parkinsonism in non-Parkinson's persons who were chronic severe heavy drinkers. This suggests that enormous alcohol excess over a long period can cause dopamine system transient problems. For the average person alcohol is not a factor to be concerned about in either the cause or long term course of Parkinson's.

Gait

Walking problems are common, disabling and a source of great frustration for Parkinson's patients. They may be related to **slowness** (bradykinesia) and respond well to medication or be secondary to **loss of balance** (postural) control which results from other basal ganglia-frontal lobe changes which do not improve with drugs. **The following may be contributing factors**: foot dystonia; hip and knee arthritis; severe disc disease; memory and thinking problems; where you are walking; and distractions such as talking. These lead to a cautious gait with loss of confidence, which can be adapted to when mild. As disability increases patients may have great problems starting to walk (especially from low chairs), get their feet tangled on turns and lose their balance. In addition patients notice that walking requires much more conscious effort and this is more difficult if thinking is slowed.

Freezing may develop and is a major problem that often responds poorly to standard antiparkinsonian therapy. Freezing appears as if the patient's feet are stuck to the floor, it lasts seconds to a minute and in addition may affect speech, writing and brushing teeth. It is more common and severe in atypical parkinsonism including progressive supranuclear palsy, vascular parkinsonism and hydrocephalus. In these disorders it responds less well to the "tricks" that are so effective in classic Parkinson's (see below). Freezing may occur as the patient starts to walk (start hesitation) when a turn is made, in a doorway, or when distracted. Patients with tremor and those who have been on selegiline are less likely to have freezing while those with more fluctuations and dyskinesias have more problems. Drug treatment is not very good but selegiline may help and increases and decreases of levodopa and dopamine agonists should be tried. With festination the patient leans forward, takes short steps, begins to almost run and frequently falls. This may be seen in the untreated patient and usually responds well to medication.

Gait problems are a major and serious component of the slowness (bradykinesia) of Parkinson's and can contribute greatly to a decline in general health. It has been clearly shown that keeping active and fit improves general health, avoids a multitude of serious problems and prolongs life. For all of these reasons Parkinson's patients, their family and health care team should make every effort to promote mobility and exercise (see section on Physiotherapy).

Tips for Initiating Movement and Walking

The following suggestions will assist you in maintaining walking and mobility. Read the entire section and **try the various "tricks" over a few days and decide which ones work for you and incorporate them into your daily routine**. Many of these involve motor and sensory cues and concentrating on paying careful attention to the action you want initiate. There is a lot of information below, you and your family and caregivers should spend time reviewing it and forming your mobility plan.

- Use a marching rhythm to move:

    - Wear a walkman with marching music and swing your arms

    - Tap the floor with your cane to a regular beat, then walk to the beat

    - Count rhythmically - one, two, three - one, two, three or vocalize something out loud

    - If not using a cane, tap your hip with your hand

- If using a walker, use one with wheels and brakes. This promotes a smoother, uninterrupted walk

- Use a laser pointer (cheap, easily available) and fix the beam about two feet in front of your feet and step over it.

• Alter your weight distribution and your direction of movement:

- Step backwards or sideways if unable to go forward

- Push down on the foot before lifting it

- Lift toes up and shift weight to back of the heels

- Stamp your feet

- Rock from side to side

- Bend knees and then straighten up

- Raise your arms in a sudden short motion and may clap your hands

- If using a cane, place it in front of your foot and try to kick it

- Use an upside-down walking stick (a cane with a straight edged handle at the bottom instead of the top). If stuck or "frozen", place this in front of your foot, close to the toes, and then step over it

- Use concentration strategies such as watching other people walk, picturing white lines on the floor to step over or focus your attention on generating large amplitude steps. Normal people do these things automatically and by concentrating, Parkinson's patients can nicely recover mobility function.

Here are some additional tips for a slow shuffling gait that causes tripping.

- Walk with a wide stance, lifting the foot forward and placing the heel down first. Make sure that your head is up and shoulders back. Look ahead instead of down and swing your arms.

- Turn by walking around in a circle, using your hands for guidance. Do not cross one foot in front of the other. Do not have your weight on the pivoting foot, as your feet will become tangled. Concentrate on walking around an arc.

- Stop and start again slowly, if you find you are moving too quickly (festination as described above).

- **Use a cane if necessary, being sure it is measured to the right height**. Correct cane height can be determined by putting your hands by your side. Stand straight; the head of the cane should be at the level of your wrist. The cane should have a rubber tip, and in winter, an ice pick. If you must grip the cane tightly for prolonged periods, the tendons in the palm may be injured, resulting in painful stiff fingers. Wrapping the handle with a soft, spongy material will help.

- **Use a walker if necessary**. Check with your doctor, nurse or physiotherapist for the one best suited for your needs. Some patients do very well with wheels on the walker and some excellent, safe, models are available. Walker with wheels are preferred for Parkinson's patients. Some types even have seats and baskets. U shaped bases give improved stability. **Walkers give a real boost to confidence and independence**. Some patients are reluctant to try a walker, most clinics have one and most patients are pleasantly surprised with their new freedom.

- Plan a simple daily routine of exercises to maintain muscle tone and coordination (see section on Physiotherapy).

- Minimize distractions and interruptions if freezing is a problem.

- Keep your cane or walker near your bed at night.

- Have your physician refer you to a physiotherapist or rehabilitation specialist for gait training and the proper use and choice of a cane or walker.

- If you tire after walking a long distance then take along a wheelchair (with attached seat).

Tips for Rising From a Chair or Bed

- Patients often have a problem with rising from a chair, couch or bed. This is a result of bradykinesia, which slows movement. **The ability to rise from a medium height, firm chair without using your hands to push up, is one of the best tests for the degree of bradykinesia**. Bradykinesia responds well to levodopa therapy.

Tips for Chair

- Move forward to the edge of the chair, then lean forward and place your feet with a wide base, firmly on the floor under your body. Use your hands on either the arm of the chair or the seat of the chair to push up into a standing position. A rocking motion or counting to 3 may help for rhythm in rising.

- Physiotherapy may be beneficial and more exercises can be prescribed for rising from a chair. Improving muscle strength will help rising (see section on Physiotherapy).

- Parkinsonian medication adjustment, especially levodopa may improve the problem.

- Avoid low and soft-cushioned chairs.

- Chairs with armrests are preferable.

- Put small (approximately 5 cm high) blocks under rear legs of chair so rising becomes easier with this forward tilt. These blocks are specially made for elevating chairs so consult your occupational therapist for more details. Make sure they are not too high or that the chair becomes unsteady.

- New "self rising" chairs are available for severely disabled patients and you might try one of the adjustable height office chairs that is comfortable (including armrests) for you.

Tips For Bed

- Sit on the side of the bed near the pillows or head of the bed so that when lying down, you are in the correct position for sleeping.

- Use a bed rope attached to the footboard of the bed. Knots should be tied along the rope for handles for the patients to pull themselves up with. The rope must be long enough to reach the patient's chest when lying down.

- Elevating the head of the bed by securing the legs on blocks makes it easier to arise.

- To avoid having to travel to the bathroom during the night, restrict fluids before bed. A bedside urinal or commode will help.

- Keep a flashlight near the bed for safety.

- Satin sheets make it easier to turn over in bed.

- For turning in bed, lie flat on back, bend knees, put your arms across chest and turn your head to the side you want to turn to. Then let your legs fall to that side and your body will follow through. It is important to note that even if you are quite disabled and have poor balance, turning in bed will usually respond to medication adjustment (see section on Sleep re night medication and upsets).

- To rise from the bed, turn onto your side, support yourself on your elbow and forearm while gripping the edge of your bed with your hands. Bend your knees up towards your chest and place your toes near the edge of the bed. Swing your feet down while pushing yourself up, first with your elbow then with your hands. Feel your head and shoulder rise as you push yourself into a sitting position. Sit on the side of the bed for sufficient time to let your blood pressure stabilize and to avoid lightheadedness and falls.

Tips for Your Family

- Offer help using a light touch to the arm or shoulder. DO NOT PUSH OR PULL.

- Step in front of your relative and ask him/her to mimic your actions. Say "follow me" and walk ahead of the patient.

- Minimize distractions and avoid interruptions when walking with the patient. For example: continue walking into the room instead of stopping at the doorway, and then turning to meet the patient. Ask the patient what distractions are most likely to cause freezing.

- Use simple, verbal commands, such as "lift right foot!", "march, left-right, left-right!" swing your arms

- Provide obstacles for your relative to step over such as pieces of paper spaced on the floor in front of him/her. If stuck try lifting the patients leg

- Remind the patient frequently about the concentration strategies discussed above.

Falls and Their Prevention

Falls are common and even patients who are only moderately affected by Parkinson's may fall. It has been shown that there is little correlation between an abnormal "pull" test and the tendency to fall. Falls result in injuries and loss of confidence and may predict subsequent nursing home admission. **Falls must be treated as a very serious problem and require detailed review**. Careful questioning about the occurrence of falls is necessary with each patient and remedial factors must be searched for. The history is most important as few patients fall in the clinic. **Risk factors include**: older age, more disability, longer duration of illness, atypical parkinsonism, impaired postural reflexes, difficulty walking and rising from a chair, dyskinesia, other neurological defects and the environment where you walk. Thirty percent of the general population over age 65 living in the community fall each year and 10% will have a serious injury. If you add Parkinson's to this, the magnitude of the problem becomes clear.

Interventions are very helpful and a detailed multidisciplinary assessment of high-risk patients who have fallen must be done. A major cause should be established in each case and remedial risk factors identified. Remedial risk factors are underdiagnosed and studies have shown that the fracture rate can be reduced by more than 50% with a detailed approach. **Hip fractures are an epidemic and falls and injury prevention strategies should be part of routine clinical practice.** Hospitals and patient societies have set up falls programs. Balance may improve with medication early in the illness but later defects involve more non-dopamine systems and respond poorly. **A home assessment by an occupational therapist for environmental factors** is very helpful, as these are the most common remedial risk factors identified. The correct footwear is important. **The most common other contributing factors are**: abnormal cardiac rhythm, postural hypotension, impaired vision, leg weakness, knee arthritis, poor balance and depression. The more risk factors the greater the fall risk.

All medication should be reviewed. The total number of drugs is directly related to the risk for falls. Sleeping medication, long acting tranquilizers, drugs for blood pressure and antidepressants are frequent contributing factors. The tricyclic drugs may be worse than the SSRI's (see section on Depression) especially if combined with cardiac medications. A careful general neurological exam should be done looking for: neck disc disease, muscle weakness, peripheral neuropathy, balance system (cerebellar) problems and signs of stroke.

Tips to Prevent Falls

Environment

- Ensure adequate lighting, especially at the top and bottom of stairs and in dark hallways. Use night-lights.

- Have your vision checked.

- Remove loose scatter rugs.

- Avoid carrying heavy objects.

- Do not leave shoes, clothing and other objects on the floor.

- Remove furniture from traffic areas.

- Remove doorsills if possible.

- Install handrails in bathroom and on stairs.

- Maintain outdoor steps and walks in good repair. Be aware of, avoid, and consider changing, uneven, slippery surfaces.

- Make sure furniture and appliances are stable.

- Normal beds and toilets tend to be too low. Toilet safety rails, a raised toilet seat, a commode chair fitted over the toilet or wooden risers may be helpful. Consult your occupational therapist or home care team for more information.

- Pets (cats and dogs) may not be advisable as they can trip you.

- A plastic bag fastened on the car seat, will make entering and exiting the car much easier.

- Do not wax bare floors.

- Wipe up liquid spills immediately.

- Install a telephone on each level of the house. Use an answering machine and set it to answer after the fourth or fifth ring to avoid rushing to the phone.

- If there is confusion, hallucinations or vivid dreams, install bed rails and seat belts for wheelchairs to avoid an unstable patient from getting up unassisted.

- Have your physician refer you to an occupational therapist for a home assessment for safety.

- Wall-to-wall carpeting will soften a fall and possibly prevent a fracture.

- Footwear

- Wear proper fitting footwear with good support.

- Keep shoes in good repair.

- Wear leather-soled shoes, as rubber or crepe grips the floor making it more difficult to walk, especially with a toe-first gait. Leather becomes smooth and slippery, so be careful on stairs.

- Strap onto your shoe or overshoe, "ice grips" which are available in health aid stores. These should be worn or carried with you in the winter.

- Women should avoid high heels.

Bathing

- Have someone with you when you bathe if you have a history of falling or unsteadiness.

- Avoid oil in the bath water.

- Use bathtub aids, such as a bath bench, table and handrails (see section on Assistive Devices and Techniques).

- Use non-slip bathtub and floor mats.

- Sit down when dressing or undressing.

- Use soap-on-a-rope to avoid bending over to pick up the soap.

- Do not lock the bathroom door. Be sure someone is within hearing distance while bathing.

Medical Tips

- **Have your doctor carefully review all the drugs your are taking**. Sleeping pills and blood pressure pills and "nerve pills" or antidepressants may be the culprit in causing more falls.

- Have your eyes checked. New glasses or cataract surgery might be needed.

- Dyskinesias could be causing the balance problems. A reduction in levodopa might help.

- Ensure that a proper diet is followed as malnutrition significantly increases the chances of falling.

- Have your blood pressure checked lying, sitting and standing.

- Sudden falls with loss of consciousness usually are related to an irregular heart rhythm (need 24-hour monitor) or postural hypotension. Ongoing low blood pressure can cause chronic unsteadiness in walking and this is often missed.

- Hip and knee arthritis and foot problems should be assessed.

Recovering From a fall

- Without someone's help: If you are on the floor on your back, use a rocking motion to turn onto your side. Use hands and push yourself up to a sitting position. Sitting up, turn slowly and come onto all fours. Walk on all fours towards a chair or heavy piece of furniture. Bring up your hands, spaced apart, on either side of the chair. Bring one knee up so the best leg is forward. Use hands to press down on the chair and then push up with the foot. Lift the hips and come up to a standing position.

- With someone's help: Again if you are on the floor on your back, use a rocking motion to turn onto your side. Use hands and push yourself up to a sitting position. Sitting up, turn slowly and come onto all fours. The person helping you should stand close with feet apart in a solid stance. Take a firm hold of the person's legs in front of you with hands spaced apart. Bring one knee up so the best leg is forward. Then slowly crawl up the person's body to their waist. The person assisting should not pull or push the patient.

These procedures should be included in an exercise program so you will be familiar with them when necessary (see section on Exercise). Because of the risk of falls, sometimes with injury, it is very important to arrange the following:

- A daily contact with a friend or relative.

- Wear a whistle, if help is within hearing distance.

- Keep a telephone or alarm system within reach from the floor.

- There are alarm systems that are connected to the telephone. A button is worn around the neck that can be pressed if emergencies arise. Contact your Parkinson's association or the Telephone Company for more information.

Exercise and Physiotherapy

The goal is to try and slow or stop the reduction in muscle strength, joint flexibility, balance and walking that occur in Parkinson's. **Preservation of function** should be the plan of action. Studies are underway to assess if physiotherapy started in the first three years after diagnosis will achieve this.

Recent studies have shown that an intensive one-month (three times per week) **physical rehabilitation program in patients with moderate disability** can give clear measurable benefit on Parkinson's scoring scales. Improvements occurred in moving from lying to standing, making a full 360 degree turn while standing, and looking over the shoulder while standing or driving. **However if exercise is not maintained the benefit is lost over six months**. An ongoing program outside the home is best as only doing exercise on one's own is difficult to maintain. The Parkinson's problems that improve most with exercise are slowness and rigidity. It has been suggested that improvement is psychological but these studies show no change in depression scales, which shows the benefit is real.

A 22 year study of healthy middle aged persons (without Parkinson's) showed a significantly reduced death rate. This is important as it also demonstrated that even modest improvements in physical fitness gave significant health benefit. It also showed a reduction in risk factors including blood pressure, body fat and lipid levels and improvement in breathing capacity and exercise cardiogram. **These results are relevant for Parkinson's patients and argue that in order to maintain overall good health any reduction in physical fitness must be vigorously opposed**. It is important to remember that Parkinson's patients are at risk, just as we all are, for the health problems that develop, as we grow older.

Parkinson's patient should commence exercising early, **before** the occurrence of muscle weakness, stooped posture, or falls. It is much more difficult to correct these problems after they start. Patients should not only carry out these exercises regularly but also attempt to continue with any other exercises or sports they enjoy. A daily walk, when weather permits, is very valuable. Physiotherapy and exercise classes are a very helpful and sociable form of activity. Tai Chi exercise helps to relax and strengthen the body and may benefit balance and coordination. It is gentle and even people unable to stand can practice it. Patients should develop a program of light to moderate exercises lasting 25 to 30 minutes, **carried out either daily or three times per week at a minimum**. You should start slowly, increase at your own rate, and stop if you become fatigued. It may take several weeks to build up your stamina.

A recent report states that high intensity resistance exercises may give up to 100 percent improvement in leg muscle weakness and physical frailty of elderly patients. Better mobility and balance were achieved and some patients became much more independent. This is very supportive of an active exercise program and shows that in addition to walking you must do some resistance training including leg and arm lifts with weights and if possible sit ups for abdominal muscles. Exercise, including walking, maintains and improves bone density and protects against the painful fractures of osteoporosis.

All the exercises listed below will help develop good body mechanics, but there are specific ones you should emphasize for particular problems. You should develop these between yourself and your clinic nurse and therapist. Shoulder and arm exercises help a frozen shoulder. Back flexibility and strength exercises can counteract stooped posture or scoliosis. Lower abdominal and pelvic exercises may help relieve constipation and urinary incontinence. **The plan should be to design the physiotherapy program to remedy the motor deficits that you have as well as to improve and maintain general fitness.**

Some specific suggestions include: **for strength**= resistance exercises; for **speed of movement**= practice; for **preparedness for movement and slowness initiating movement**= repetition and rhythmic activities and cuing; for **sequential movements**= simple sequences and large amplitude movements. Also note that karate improves fast movements and there are specific exercises for truncal stiffness. Reduced muscle mass impairs balance and exercise can avoid and improve the shortness of breath that some patients develop.

Many Parkinson's patients have bothersome hip and knee arthritis. Regular moderate exercise, either walking (aerobic) or weights and stretching (resistance) can relieve pain and improve function. This requires dedicated effort of 30 minutes at least three times per week.

Patients with more advanced Parkinson's may find some of the exercises difficult or impossible. If so, you should review them and concentrate on those you can do. If you have other problems, such as heart disease, consult your physician about the level of activity best for you.

Therefore in summary: a continuing exercise program has been shown in studies to be a very important factor in

maintaining and improving a patient's level of function. The program must be done regularly as benefits are lost if exercise is stopped.

Tips for Exercise

- Wear comfortable, loose-fitting clothing. Tracksuits are very popular.

- Exercise with a companion or join a group. It makes it more fun and will benefit you both.

- Exercise to music. Use either your own or exercise cassettes available from the Parkinson's or physiotherapy clinics.

- Exercise at the same time every day and when your medications are working at their peak.

- Start your program slowly and progress gradually over a period of weeks.

- Do all exercises slowly in a relaxed, gentle and consistent manner.

- Never bounce on a "stretch." Feel the stretch and hold it, working up from 3 to 5 or 10 seconds.

- Work up to 5 or 10 repetitions of each exercise.

- Develop a plan for yourself using the advice of a physiotherapist and the suggestions outlined in this section. Decide what your major problems are and give them special attention in addition to a general program.

Home Exercise Program

Repeat each exercise three times

While Sitting or Standing

1. FACE

    a. Raise your eyebrows and wrinkle your forehead.

    b. Open your mouth as wide as possible.

    c. Blow out your cheeks.

    d. Try to whistle.

    e. Wriggle your nose.

    f. Smile, frown and smile again.

2. NECK (Done slowly in a relaxed manner)

    a. Tuck in your chin and place your finger on it. Draw your neck and head backwards (away from finger) as far as possible (do not tilt your head backward). Hold for 5 seconds. Return to a relaxed position. Repeat.

    b. Look straight down, putting your chin on your chest. Hold for 5 seconds. Return to a relaxed position. Repeat.

    c. Turn your head to the right, looking over right shoulder. Return your head to center, looking straight ahead. Repeat three times.

    d. Turn your head to the left repeat three times.

    e. Tilt your head to the right, bringing your right ear close to your shoulder (do not raise your shoulder). Hold for 5 seconds, then return head to the upright position, looking straight ahead. Repeat three times. Tilt your head to the left, bringing left ear close to shoulder. Hold for five seconds. Return to the upright position. Repeat three times.

3. HAND AND WRIST

    a. Hold your arms, relaxed, out to your sides.

    b. Move your hands up and down 5 times.

    c. Move your hands side to side 5 times.

    d. Rotate your hands in circles 5 times clockwise and 5 times counterclockwise. Lower arms.

    e. Stretch your hands and fingers out straight. Relax.

    f. Squeeze your hands into fists. Relax.

    g. Spread your fingers apart, keeping them as straight as possible. Hold for 5 seconds, then bring them together. Repeat three times.

    h. Practice picking up coins and small objects from a table.

4. SHOULDER

    a. Hold onto opposite elbows to form "a cradle." Lift cradle straight up over your head, then back down.

    b. Rock cradle from side to side.

    c. Move cradle in large circles, first in one direction, then the other.

    d. With arms straight down, shrug shoulders up to ears. Return to a relaxed position.

    e. Raise your right arm straight up. Bend your right elbow

so that your hand is hanging relaxed behind your back. Raise your left arm straight up. Bend arm to grasp right elbow with left hand. Push right elbow slowly and gently backwards. Return to a relaxed position. Switch arms and repeat.

While Standing (stand with your feet your shoulder width apart)

1. SHOULDER STRETCH

Clasp your hands together behind your back. Keeping your elbows and back straight, gently raise arms upward. Return to a relaxed position. Repeat.

2. BACK FLEXIBILITY (if your balance is unsteady, have someone standing by or hold onto a chair)

   a. Corner stretch - stand facing a corner with one hand on each wall at shoulder height. Move your chest (not chin) towards the corner. Hold for 10 to 15 seconds. Return to a relaxed position. Repeat a few times with your hands at different heights.

   b. Stooped posture exercises - stand with your back against a wall. Press your shoulders and the small of your back against the wall. Stretch your arms to each side so that the backs of your hands are touching the wall. Slide your hands up the wall above your head, keeping arms and upper body against the wall. Return to a relaxed position. Repeat three times. Raise your right leg out in front of you as high as possible. Return to a relaxed position. Repeat with left leg. Move away from the wall and walk with your arms clasped behind your back. Return to a relaxed position. Repeat.

c. Side stretch - raise your arms above your head and clasp hands together. Slowly bend to the side and slightly forward until you feel a gentle stretch. Hold for three breaths. Straighten up and repeat to the other side.

d. Foreword stretch - place your hands on your hips. Gently keeping your back straight, bend forward from the waist until you feel your weight transferring to the balls of your feet (no more than 20 degrees from the vertical), hold for 3 seconds and then straighten up. Repeat.

e. Backward stretch - place your hands on the small of your back, just below your waist. Slowly bend backwards, as far as you can comfortably go. Hold for 3 seconds and then straighten up. Repeat.

f. Back rotation - place your hands on your hips. Rotate your back to the right by looking back over your right shoulder and rotating your back to follow. Make sure your left shoulder comes forward. Hold for 3 seconds. Repeat on left side.

g. Unsteady gait exercise - begin walking by lifting your right foot forward and placing the heel down first. Swing your left arm forward at the same time. Keep your head up, your shoulders back and look straight ahead, not down. Repeat using your left foot and right arm, keeping your feet apart. Continue walking in this pattern and concentrate on swinging your arms.

While Sitting (use a hard straight-backed chair)

1. SINGLE ARM STRETCH - keeping the elbow straight, stretch your right arm over your head as high as possible. Return to a relaxed position. Repeat with left arm.

2. TRUNK TWIST WITH ARM STRETCH - stretch your right arm out to the side with the palm facing back. Slowly twist your head, right shoulder and arm, and body to the right. Turn as far as is comfortable. Hold for 5 seconds. Return to a relaxed position. Repeat on your left side.

3. HIP STRETCH - Sit sideways on the chair with your right arm resting comfortably on the back of the chair and your left hip on the forward edge of the seat. With your left arm, raise your left knee to your chest and then lower the leg and stretch it back behind you as far as you comfortably can. Repeat 3 to 5 times. Reverse your position and repeat with your right leg.

4. HAMSTRING STRETCH - Sit in the chair with your right foot on the floor and your left foot resting on a chair or table of equal height to the one you are sitting on. Keeping your left leg straight and your arms stretched out in front, gently bend forward from the waist until a comfortable stretch is felt. Hold for 3 to 5 seconds. Return to a relaxed position. Repeat with your left foot on the floor and right foot on the chair or table.

5. LEG AND ANKLE STRETCHES

    a. Straighten out your right leg and hold for 5 seconds. Return to a relaxed position. Repeat three times. Repeat with left leg.

b. Starting with your feet flat on the floor, raise your bent right knee up and then lower your foot onto the floor. Repeat three times. Relax and repeat with your left knee.

c. Extend and flex your right ankle, as in the flutter kick. Repeat three times. Repeat with left ankle.

d. Make large circles with your right foot. Repeat with left foot.

While Lying on Your Back

Your should use a firm comfortable surface such as a carpeted floor or a firm bed. Use a small cushion to support your head and neck. During the exercises, try to keep the small of your back pressed against the surface. Discontinue the exercises should they cause, or aggravate, back pain.

1. PELVIC TILT - Bend your knees and place feet flat on the surface you are lying on. Push the small of your back down onto the surface by tightening the lower abdomen. Hold for 3 to 5 seconds. Relax and repeat. Raise your hips off the surface. Hold for 3 to 5 seconds. Relax and repeat.

2 UPPER ABDOMINALS - Bend your knees and place your feet flat on the surface. Flatten your back against the surface as in the pelvic tilt. Reach your arms over your knees and pull your shoulder blades up from the surface. Hold for 3 to 5 seconds. Return to a relaxed position. Repeat.

3. OBLIQUE ABDOMINALS - Lie as in the pelvic tilt. Reach both arms slowly to the right to the outside of your knees, raising your head and shoulder blades off the surface. Hold for 3 to 5 seconds. Return to a relaxed position. Repeat to the left of your knees.

4. FRONT THIGH STRETCH - Bend your knees. Keeping the small of your back pressed against the surface, grasp your right knee and bring it up to your chest. Stretch your left leg out and press it against the surface. Hold for 3 to 5 seconds. Return to a relaxed position. Repeat with left knee and right leg.

5. BACK THIGH STRETCH - Stretch your arms above your head. Raise your right knee. Straighten out the right leg and stretch your heel to the ceiling. Point your toes toward the ceiling. Bend the knee and place your foot on the surface. Return to a relaxed position. Repeat with the left knee.

6. BACK STRETCH AND RELAXATION - Lie with your legs out straight and your arms at your sides, palms facing up. Flatten your back to the surface. Try and relax, letting the muscles stretch to allow your arms and legs to straighten out. Breathe deeply and relax for 5 to 15 minutes.

While Lying on Your Side

1. SIDE LEG RAISES FOR THIGHS, HIPS AND WAIST - lie on your right side, resting your head comfortably on your extended right arm. Place your left hand on the surface at waist level to maintain your balance. Bend your right leg. Keeping your left leg straight and toes pointed forward, slowly raise and lower the leg. Repeat 3 to 5 times. Turn over onto left side and repeat.

2. HIP EXERCISES

    a. Lying on your right side with right leg slightly bent, raise your left leg about 30 degrees and move it forward in front of you, keeping it straight. Hold for 5 seconds. Return to a relaxed position. Repeat 3 to 5 times.

b. Lying on right side, cross your left leg over your right to rest on surface in front of you. Keeping your right leg comfortably straight, raise it towards the ceiling keeping toes pointed forward. Hold for 5 seconds and relax slowly. Repeat 3 to 5 times.

c. Turn over on left side and repeat a. and b.

While Lying on Your Stomach (place a small pillow under your abdomen for comfort)

1. ARM LIFTS FOR STOOPED POSTURE - Stretch your arms on the surface in front of your head. Raise your right arm as high as possible and turn your head to look at it. Lower your arm. Raise your left arm and turn your head to look at it. Repeat 3 to 5 times.

2. LEG STRENGTHENING EXERCISE - Resting your head comfortably on your folded arms, raise your right leg about six inches above the surface, keeping the knee as straight as possible. Lower leg slowly. Repeat with left leg. Repeat exercise 3 to 5 times.

3. KNEE EXERCISE - Bend your right knee up as far as possible towards your buttock, keeping your thigh on the surface. Hold for 3 to 5 seconds and straighten out slowly. Repeat 3 to 5 times. Repeat with left knee.

Passive Exercises

For the patient who has long periods of immobility, gentle passive exercises, where another person moves the patient's limbs, can help to prevent stiff muscles and joints and promote comfort. The helper simply lifts and moves the arms, legs and neck in gentle movements that imitate normal actions. These can be taught be a physiotherapist.

1. Raise both of the patient's arms above the head and lower them.

2. Straighten the patient's legs out when sitting.

3. Turn the patient's head gently from side to side.

4. Lower the patient's head gently down towards the chest and raise it back up.

5. Note: Do not attempt the following unless the helper is confident that they themselves will not fall and the patient has no history of falling. Stand in front of the sitting patient. Brace your feet firmly, with your toes touching the patient's, to avoid slipping. Grasping the patient's hands, raise the patient to a standing position. Raise the patient's arms above the head. Lower the patient back down.

For more information on exercises, see section on Movement Problems. As well, the section on Shortness of Breath contains breathing exercises.

Scoliosis

As the disability progresses, patients frequently develop **a lean to one side**. For most patients this is quite minor but deserves attention as progression may be slowed and even if minor it may add to balance loss. X-ray studies have shown that there are usually multiple spinal curves with an overall tilt to one side. Sometimes this becomes quite severe and impairs balance and leads to more falls. There is no relation between the side of onset of symptoms and the side of leaning.

Treatment is difficult. The withdrawal of dopamine agonists is occasionally of short-term benefit. An exercise program may be helpful as outlined below and should be initiated early to see if progression can be prevented (discuss first with your physician or physiotherapist). Spinal corrective surgery has been done in some patients. This is very major surgery and should be done infrequently and only after careful consideration.

A severe forward bend when standing is seen rarely and has a variable response to levodopa. It is worse in "off" periods and with fatigue. Response to treatment is not satisfactory.

Exercises for Scoliosis

- Lying on your stomach. Keeping your right leg straight, lift it toward the ceiling. At the same time, raise your left arm and hold for 5 seconds. Return to a relaxed position. Repeat with left leg and right arm

- Standing beside a wall. With the side you lean to closest to the wall, place your feet about 10 inches out from it. Raise your wall side arm above your head. Push your hip against the wall with outside arm against the wall for balance.

- Sitting or standing with a large towel. Place your right arm over your right shoulder and your left arm behind your back. Grasp towel in both hands. Pull towel up and down 5 times, as if drying your back. Return to a relaxed position. Reverse arms and repeat.

- When sitting try and sit straight. It is not clear if a brace will help or be uncomfortable. You should ask an expert such as an experienced physiotherapist, rehabilitation physician or orthopedist.

- Patients with a forward bend should concentrate on standing straight (hard to maintain), exercising back extension (hold you straight) muscles.

Hand Deformity

Some patients with longstanding advanced disability may develop hand deformities. These problems seem less frequent in the past few years with better drug therapy. Some of these are related to chronic nerve compression in the back of the upper arm (radial nerve at the triceps muscle level), often related to poor wheelchair position and appear as a flexed hand (wrist drop). This can be prevented with attention to bed and wheel chair position and use of padding and pillows. Other patients develop severe flexion of the fingers into the palm that causes chronic skin infection and makes the hand less functional. This problem may be helped with tendon release surgery but early use of splints and careful skin care will often avoid surgery.

Hospital Care Including Surgery

In hospital care for patients with Parkinson's gives many opportunities for problems. With careful attention to detail **most can be avoided and the patient will be spared much discomfort**. At home patients and their caregivers have organized their daily plan often with things happening every hour. Hospitals do not work this way and both parties will have to work together for the best care for the patient.

Confusion and delirium can quickly occur when the patient is out of the home environment, ill and receiving new treatment for the problem that required admission. Six risk factors have been identified and if they are carefully attended to, many episodes of delirium will be prevented. **The risk factors are: memory loss; sleep deprivation; immobility; visual impairment; hearing impairment; and dehydration**. The prevention strategy is called the Elder Life Program. It can be tailored to individual risk factors and includes: frequent reorientation and mentally stimulating activities; three times daily ambulation or other exercises; visual aids and hearing devices; careful attention to hydration; and adequate sleep without drugs by taking a warm drink a bedtime, back massage, relaxation tapes and music and attention to a quiet ward environment. **These treatment adjustments are simple and family can help**. The concept is prevention, a geriatrician or internist is most likely to give you advice.

Receiving medication on time is very important for Parkinson's patients. For surgery, levodopa and dopamine agonists may **be given up to four hours before surgery** and sometimes even a little closer. Recent anesthesia guidelines indicated that two hours restriction for liquid and six hours for solids was a good plan. Some Parkinson's patients have delayed stomach emptying and this should be considered. If really necessary a chewed tablet of Sinemet with a small amount of water two hours before anesthesia may safely give great relief. Anticholinergics should be slowly removed prior to surgery, especially abdominal surgery, as they may cause impairment in intestinal motility. Patients taking selegiline should discontinue use 10 days prior to major surgery. Demerol (meperidine) should not be used in Parkinson's. It has caused acute parkinsonism and also severe high blood pressure has occurred if it is taken with selegiline. It is reassuring to remember that patients may be off levodopa for up to a week before their disability worsens significantly.

Patients who are going to have major abdominal surgery may not be able to take oral medication for a week or more. For these patients and indeed **for all Parkinson's patients having surgery there should be careful planning and many serious problems and much patient discomfort can be avoided**. Avoiding marked worsening of Parkinson's with proper medication management can prevent chest infections and leg vein thrombosis. Pulmonary function should be formally tested if the patient has moderate or greater disability (see section on Respiratory Problems). It is best to have surgery in the morning and early in the week when specialist help is more available.

The Toronto Parkinson's clinic group has described a very good drug schedule using apomorphine by injection and suppositories of domperidone. This requires planning before surgery. The patient's dose of apomorphine is established (1-2mg every 1-3 hours) and domperidone 20 mg by mouth is given for three days before surgery. After operation apomorphine is started and domperidone rectal suppositories (60 mg 3 times daily) are given. If domperidone is not available then metoclopramide (Maxeran) is NOT a safe alternative. Sublingual apomorphine may be useful in future.

Following the operation, **antiparkinsonian drugs should resume as soon as the patient can swallow**. The exception is selegiline, which should be restarted several days later.

Every attempt should be made to mobilize the patient early. Some rare blood pressure changes have occurred with some anaesthetics (cyclopropane and halothane). **Bring at least one day's supply and a written list of times and dosages of your medication to the hospital**. Any experimental drugs and information regarding the study should be brought with you and given to the nursing staff.

A malignant hyperthermia-like illness is a risk when dopamine stimulants are withdrawn. The symptoms are: fever, sweating, increased rigidity and tremor, reduced consciousness and swallowing, rapid heart rate and blood pressure changes. The risk is higher in more disabled patients and this is a very serious problem that should be managed in intensive care with fluids, restarting dopamine drugs, sedation with minor tranquilizers and dantrolene and bromocriptine for rigidity. Drugs that block dopamine receptors, major tranquilizers and metoclopramide can both cause and worsen the condition.

Patients may become confused and have hallucinations after surgery (see prevention in this section). Drugs must be carefully reviewed. Drugs for pain are needed but will worsen confusion when used in addition to the antiparkinson drugs. Anticholinergic drugs are often given after prostate surgery and may cause confusion (see section on Memory Disorders). Ondansetron (Zofran), a serotonin blocking drug, is available for intravenous use and has been used in some patients.

Humour

Mother Nature gave us humour to lighten the load. Unfortunately, the requirement of our egos to take ourselves too seriously inhibits our use of this marvellous tool to relieve our anxieties. Humour serves to put everything in perspective. The best comedians poke good fun at our many failings, and usually the recipients enjoy the pokes as much as the rest of the audience. Humour may help create a positive outlook and improve self-esteem. Humour, as a reliever of stress has proven medical benefits, including muscle relaxation and the release of endorphins which are the body's natural painkillers. A few light-hearted cracks, a good comedy show, funny card or note in the mail, can do much to "lighten the load" for patient, caregiver and treatment team.

Tips for Humour

• Rent funny movies such as the old Marx Brothers or Charlie Chaplin favorites, Monty Python, A Fish Called Wanda, Patch Adams or Mr. Bean.

• Watch the comedy shows on television including great reruns of Cheers and Seinfeld and the late night comedy shows. Many of these are worth recording and watching later.

Employment

Many Parkinson's patients are young and still employed. With some adjustments and support of family and co-workers, patients can continue working. This of course not only gives financial benefits, but also enhances feelings of independence and self-worth. With good medication management and support, many of our patients have enjoyed long and productive work time in the years after diagnosis.

Tips for Employment

- Inform your employer and co-workers that you have Parkinson's. This will prevent any obvious symptoms from being misinterpreted.

- Discuss with your physician the timing of your medication to cover more stressful hours of work.

- Request a referral to an occupational therapist to discuss techniques and equipment to make tasks easier.

- To improve writing difficulties make use of computers, typewriters, dictaphones, and pen or pencil grips.

- Discuss with your employer the possibility of reduced or flexible hours or a transfer to less demanding work.

- If you become unable to work, be very aware of your disability coverage and pension before any final decisions are made. Discuss this both with company human resources people and someone outside.

- Never accept termination or layoff if it is not to your advantage.

Estrogen

The incidence of Parkinson's is slightly less in females and the question has been raised as to whether **estrogen is a protective factor**. Recent studies have shown that estrogen decreases striatal dopamine breakdown (by reducing COMT gene activity) and therefore making more dopamine available just as COMT inhibitors do (see section on COMT inhibitors). It is possible that this dopamine sparing effect is the reason for the lower incidence and some of the other benefits described below but much more study is needed.

Postmenopausal estrogen therapy may have a beneficial effect on memory in women with Parkinson's and its use has been associated with a reduced risk of Parkinson's with memory loss and also of Alzheimer's. One small study showed that women who took estrogen after menopause were less likely to develop Parkinson's but this needs more study before it can be stated that estrogen reduces the risk. It has now been clearly shown those women on estrogen before levodopa is needed **have milder** Parkinson's.

The use of estrogen in female Parkinson's patients causes no worsening of motor activity and transdermal use may even give slight benefit. **Therefore estrogen is well tolerated and may even help some female patients**. Men with prostate cancer have been treated with estrogen preparations for many years with no worsening of Parkinson's. The effect of estrogen on brain cells and nerve growth factors is an area of intense research activity and a number of other positive effects have recently been shown (see section on Osteoporosis).

Pregnancy

There are less than 40 pregnancies reported in Parkinson's patients but despite this **small experience some helpful guidelines and information are available**. Animal studies have shown the following: levodopa has caused some fetal abnormalities including low birth weight and liver, heart and bone problems. Pergolide, bromocriptine and pramipexole seem safe. Ropinerole may cause reduced survival and digit abnormalities. Selegiline has caused problems and amantadine clearly causes malformations.

Human experience shows that Parkinson's may worsen during pregnancy and improve after delivery. Therefore if a patient is already on antiparkinson medication stopping it may not be a good option. Levodopa use during pregnancy has not been associated with any major maternal or baby problems. Bromocriptine has been widely used to facilitate pregnancy in women with prolactin disorders (who did not have Parkinson's) and in at least one Parkinson's patient and all was well. There is similar but smaller non-Parkinson's experience with pergolide. Pramipexole use has not as yet been reported in human pregnancy and the manufacturer recommends caution however the animal studies have shown no problems. Major birth defects have been reported with amantadine and there is no experience with selegiline and neither of these two drugs should be used.

Breast feeding is quite feasible while on antiparkinson therapy. Dopamine agonists inhibit lactation and probably should not be used. Amantadine is in very low amounts in breast milk and no infant problems are reported. It is not known if selegiline is excreted in breast milk. Levodopa appears in breast milk and levels of both regular and slow release preparations peak at about three hours and return to baseline at six hours. It is in low concentration in breast milk and the dose the infant receives is very small and no problems are reported.

Combining the animal and human experience the following general guidelines can be offered:

- The question of pregnancy and parkinsonism should be discussed in detail with your physicians and this should include stage, exact diagnosis and prognosis. This would best be done before pregnancy

- It must be remembered the overall human experience with Parkinson's in pregnancy is small and you must access the best sources of information.

- Parkinson's may worsen during pregnancy.

- Do not stop any drug suddenly.

- Amantadine and selegiline should not be used during pregnancy, amantadine is probably safe for the nursing mother and infant.

- Dopamine agonist use during pregnancy seems safe because of the extensive use of bromocriptine during pregnancy in non-Parkinsons (and one patient with Parkinson's).

- There is no human experience with pramipexole, and ropinerole should not be used because of abnormalities in the animal studies.

- Dopamine agonists may reduce lactation but some mothers have nursed while on them.

- Levodopa is probably safe in pregnancy but the animal experience suggests some caution and it seems best avoided if possible. Levodopa is safe for the nursing infant.

From the above one is left with the following; do not take amantadine or selegiline during pregnancy; avoid levodopa if possible (may use when nursing) and dopamine agonists (for bromocriptine see 6 and 7 above) are safe in pregnancy. A reasonable approach may be to use bromocriptine during pregnancy and levodopa after.

The decision for pregnancy is best made with the prospective parents and physician, weighing the patient's desires and illness, the future and the variable but often mild course of Parkinson's in younger patients. The joy of child rearing can be fully appreciated by the parents with big doses of humor, mutual support and understanding and clear honest explanation to the child. The child should be made helpful and independent as early as possible without overburdening the child or older siblings. Show hope and optimism not sadness and self-pity. With a positive family approach your children will be well equipped to handle other crises in life. As one Parkinson's mother reported: you will be rewarded with comments like; "Mom does not smile as much as before (because of reduced facial expression) but she always smiles in her heart."

Patient Services

Most patients and their families at one time or another will need help in coping with the problems and complexities of this long-term disability. When problems arise, feel free to discuss them with your doctor or nurse so that the appropriate referrals may be made to the many available community services. These services allow patients to live at home longer and help improve their quality of life. They also provide needed relief to the caregivers. Many of these services are covered under medical insurance plans. The following is a list of services available in most communities.

Home Care

A program to satisfy the need for professional health care at home. Your doctor will refer you to Home Care if it is needed. A coordinator will interview you in your home and then make a referral to the appropriate service needed. Services supplied include: nursing, physiotherapy, occupational therapy, speech therapy, social work, nutritional counseling, homemaking and respiratory care.

Meals on Wheels

Delivers 3 meals in the morning, 5 days a week to people who are unable to prepare their own meals. The meals come ready for heating.

Professional Homemaking Services

These homemakers will come to the home to assist people who wish to continue to live on their own. They provide help with shopping, some housekeeping, preparing meals, and personal care. This service can be covered by provincial insurance if done through Home Care.

Day Hospital Programs

These programs provide care and treatment in a hospital setting to disabled persons during the day, a few days per week, depending on the need. This allows the patient to maintain daily activities and receive rehabilitation and support services. Also the caregiver is given assistance and some free time from looking after the patient at home. Some of our patients who are not doing well and who have multiple medical problems in addition to parkinsonism, have received help from short-term admission to a geriatric assessment unit. During admission, the need for each drug can be evaluated and the whole patient and treatment program can be assessed.

Respite Care Programs

Respite care allows the patient and caregiver to both have a vacation away from each other. The patient may spend, for example one month in a hospital or lodge and then two months at home. This varies between shorter and longer periods and can even be planned for at the same time each year.

Permanent Placement

Permanent placement homes can be found in the directory of resources in your community. These are usually in the form of nursing homes, homes for the aged and chronic care hospitals that provide a supervised caring environment. Waiting lists are long so the need must be anticipated and acted upon before it becomes critical. Home care programs often assist in finding the appropriate facility.

Transportation Services

Special transportation services are available for those who cannot drive or take a bus because of a disability. Applications are available at the city transportation service and have to be signed by your doctor. Handicap stickers are also available for cars carrying disabled persons. These stickers allow parking in the "handicap only" zones and can be obtained at your local motor vehicle registration unit. Your doctor must sign an application form available at the unit.

Parkinson's Associations

These associations offer information, education and support to patients, their family and friends. Specifically, they can provide information on income tax deductions, drug benefit plans, assistive devices, social services and other benefits. These societies also raise money for research and patient care. They are a very important component of the total care program for patients. Every Parkinson's family should belong to their local organization. **The Parkinson's Society of Ottawa-Carleton** functions at a very high level and an outline of their many activities is described below.

- individual counseling
- support groups for people with Parkinson's, caregivers, family members and couples
- education workshops
- physiotherapy classes
- information sharing through a resource centre and newsletter
- social events
- family physician education programs

They can be contacted for further information at:

Parkinson's Society of Ottawa-Carleton
1053 Carling Ave
Ottawa, Ontario K1Y 4E9
Tel: (613)722-9238 | Fax: (613)722-3241
Internet:http://www.ncf.carleton.ca/freeport/social.services/
parkinson/menu

Directory of Resources for Senior Citizens

Senior citizens are not the only ones who will benefit from this directory. The directory is similar to a phone book only it provides some detail about each service. This type of informative book can be obtained through the senior citizen council in your area.

Assistive Devices and Techniques

In the course of their daily activities, patients can experience a variety of difficulties. Many assistive devices and techniques have been developed to assist in handling them. Support agencies are familiar with this equipment and can advise patients on its purchase and use. Your physician may refer you to an occupational therapist who can teach you how to use these devices as well as how to conserve your energy and time. Most items are readily available from medical and health supply stores, and there may be government programs available to assist in their purchase. **Patients and families should go to these stores and browse**. There are amazing and ingenious aids available. In addition, imaginative use of normal household implements, supplemented by a little ingenuity, and hammer and saw, can often produce simple inexpensive solutions. If such equipment, purchased or homemade, can help you maintain your independence, then it is well worth the investment.

Dressing

- Use velcro fasteners and zippers if buttoning of shirts and pants is a problem. Just remove previous buttons and replace with velcro strips.

- Elastic shoe laces - where elastic replaces the shoestring. Instead of tying your shoes, a loop at the end of the elastic is slipped over a hook at the top of the shoe. So to take your shoe off and the loop is just unhooked.

- Track or sweat suits make dressing more comfortable and simpler.

- A dressing stick or cane makes it easier to pull up pants and underwear.

- Long shoe horns and long handled reaching tongs are available.

Bathroom

- Elevated toilet seat.

- Safety handles around the toilet seat.

- Handrails or grab bars for the bathtub and non-slip mats.

- Special chairs designed for the bathtub or shower.

- Foam rubber handle grips for gripping toothbrush or utensil.

- Soap-on-a-rope or in a dispensable bottle.

- Shower hose for the person who cannot bend over or who needs to be seated in the shower or bath.

- Long handled brush or sponge for washing below the knees.

- Electric razors or toothbrushes make these chores easier and more effective.

- Wash mitts or terry cloth gloves eliminate the need for a washcloth.

Bedroom

- Satin sheets allow easier movement in bed.

- Wooden blocks to elevate the bed and make it easier to get in and out of bed.

- A bed rope attached to the footboard of the bed. Knots should be tied along the rope for handles for the patients to pull themself up with. The rope must be long enough to reach the patient's chest when lying down.

- Commode for the bedroom at night.

Eating

- Clip-on ring to provide an edge for the plate. This prevents food from being pushed off the plate.

- Rocker knife for cutting with one hand. It also has parts on the tip to be used as a fork.

- Insulated drinking cups with openings in the cover to prevent spills and keep the fluid warm for a longer period.

- Warming trays to keep food from getting cold while you eat.

Home Making

- "Extend your reach" handles for dusting and cleaning up spills.

- Long handled dust pan.

- Aprons with large pockets to free hands for walker or cane.

- Spray hose attachment for rinsing dishes and vegetables.

- "Lazy Susan" (revolving turntable) kept on the kitchen counter to store supplies within easy reach.

Travel

Patients with very significant disabilities may travel quite well. Patients are strongly encouraged to travel. Most patients who travel south in the winter feel better in the warmer climate and in addition the bright days are part of light therapy and help relieve depression. Do not curtail this stress-relieving activity because of fear of travelling.

Tips for Travel

- A letter from your doctor stating your medical problems should be obtained. A letter for your medication may be needed to clear customs.

- Check health insurance. You may need extra travel health insurance to cover cash payments out of the country. Carry your provincial health care and private supplemental insurance information with you. It is wise to make duplicates of these important papers.

- Find the name and address of a neurologist or general practitioner who practices at your travel destination. Your doctor or a friend already living in the area can help with this.

- Prebook your airline (or train) seat and explain your disabilities for extra service. Bulkhead seats may give less leg room but are more private. Many planes have seats in the first cabin just across from a washroom.

- Wheelchairs are available and airline personnel are very helpful and know the shortcuts around the airport.

- Travel by car and bus can also be favourable if the trip is carefully planned with shorter drives and more stopovers.

- Bring enough medication for the holiday. Your home prescriptions cannot be filled when out of province or the country. **Know and record the generic names of all your drugs** (for example levodopa-carbidopa=Sinemet) in case you lose your drugs or require hospital admission. The drugs are available in other countries with different brand names.

- Carry your medication with you. Do not put it in your checked luggage. Bring extra medication and consider splitting it into two sets in case of loss.

- For overnight flights you may want to continue with your every 3-4 hour levodopa doses as you do in the daytime.

- Leg and foot swelling (edema) is common during long air travel. You should wear loose fitting shoes (preferably with laces). Move your legs frequently when sitting, flex and extend your feet. Get up and move about if possible. Try and elevate your legs as much as possible. Use only small amounts of alcohol. All of these points will avoid phlebitis, which is a risk with prolonged immobility.

- Check the location of the hospital and other medical facilities upon arrival, in case of emergency.

Coping With the Illness

This section will address: caring for patients with chronic illness; quality of life for caregivers and patient; caregiver burden; and some general patient and caregiver concerns. **It has been shown that patients with chronic illnesses like**

Parkinson's often do not receive adequate medical care for their non-Parkinson's medical problems. The feeling seems to be that if the primary illness is well treated then all the others are secondary. It is the "it's all your Parkinson's" brush off and this is not acceptable. A question asked on every visit should be **"what is your main problem today?"** The answers are often very different from what the nurse and doctor suspect is the problem to focus on first. **The aim is to have active management of chronic illness** and there are specific programs now that involve nurses and primary care physicians but you must be careful it is not just a "for profit" run program. Those who are fortunate enough to have a Parkinson's clinic that they can attend will get the proper advice there. But even then you must take care to have your general health needs fully assessed and treated considering the thoughts above. **Your best management plan is to have a family physician or internist who knows you and your problems well**. Only 15% of Parkinson's patients are admitted to hospital for Parkinson's only. The rest have general medical conditions including: chest infections; bladder problems; surgical conditions; other neurological problems; and falls. An optimistic note is that Parkinson's patients have a lower risk of cancer.

Patients have long been aware of the **quality of their life since they became ill** and this is now a major focus of care programs. It has been shown that interventions to improve the physical and mental state of patients, improves that of both the caregiver and patient and this is a **powerful argument to fully address the whole patient and those helping**. Scales to measure quality of life have been developed for both patient and caregiver. Other studies show that treating depression and mobility problems gives the caregiver great relief. The depressed patient with memory loss adds much more burden than the patient with mobility problems only. Caregiver strain and depression increase as the patient worsens and caregivers often have their own health problems and physical limitations. The use of assessment scales for these issues is important because various interventions to try and improve things can be evaluated. **Problems must be identified early and appropriate steps initiated.**

Some of the programs available are: respite care both in and outside the home; in-home caregiver training; and adult day care. Peer and group support is important, it reduces stress and depression by exposure to other people with the same burdens. This is an opportunity to exchange ideas, reduce social isolation, share information on available resources, dispel misconceptions and foster self-confidence. There are also educational/counseling programs which differ from support groups in that the focus is on education such as teaching problem solving or coping skills and this lowers caregiver strain by being more prepared for new challenges that will occur.

Chronic disabilities of movement, such as Parkinson's, with their slowness, tremor and multiple other problems can be tough, depressing and demoralizing for the patient and family. Patients must struggle with the self-image problems of having the illness, their loss of independence in work and recreation and all of the small nuisances that develop over the years of the illness. Loved ones suffer part of this with the patient, plus the additional upset of seeing a parent or partner disabled, the feelings of inadequacy and guilt that often develop, and the changes in their own life that are required to look after the patient. **To handle all this requires insight, an understanding, positive attitude and a unified effort by the patient, friends, family and treatment team**. The clinic team and neurologist must identify caregiver strain and make an appropriate referral. If there is medical uncertainty then it is wonderful to hear your doctor say "we will work on it together". **Caring is the chief ingredient of patient management.**

The reduced facial expression, that is part of Parkinson's, often makes it difficult to interpret a patient's emotional responses. Patients and those interacting with them should be aware of this. Patients should make people aware of their feelings and try to compensate for this. Those talking to patients should realize that this is not always a sign of sadness or depression and that the patient may really be very interested in, or find humorous, the story you are telling them.

When in public, patients are concerned about what others will think of them. This and other stressful social situations will increase rigidity or tremor and may be improved with counseling, stress management sessions and relaxation therapy. Caregivers will also benefit from these psychological therapies. Knowledge and understanding of the disability and its complications will help the patient and caregiver cope with day to day trials. **Parkinson's associations, support groups and exercise classes, can be of major benefit in providing information, understanding, advice and positive feedback.**

Tips for the Patient

- Take one day at a time.

- Don't dwell on the long-term outlook of the illness. Every patient is different.

- Educate yourself and learn as much as possible about the disability, progression, treatment and research.

- Try to keep as independent as possible.

- Be cheerful and optimistic.

- Focus on and make the most of small benefits.

- Thank those who are looking after you frequently. They are not having much fun either and your thanks will help them cope.

- Physiotherapy and speech therapy may help in adapting to, and improving certain aspects of the disability.

- Occupational therapy can be useful in assessing the home for the use of aids such as handrails in the bathroom, aids in the kitchen or other assistive devices.

- Learn to delegate your responsibilities if you are unable to accomplish them or find them frustrating.

- Remain active. Your body will tell you if the activity is stressful and if a less strenuous activity is necessary. Exercise will help you maintain your level of function.

- Pace your activities. Set aside time for daily rest if you tire more easily.

- Maintain your social life even if it becomes more limited or if new activities are needed.

- Try to overcome feelings of embarrassment when with others or when in public. Admit to having Parkinson's. People will respond to your own secure self-image. Remember many well people are very uncomfortable with illness. Your attitude can influence them.

- Patients with a positive attitude do better and so do their caregivers.

- Mention and seek help and advice for the small nuisance things that are bothering you.

- It has been shown the close feelings and positive aspects of your relationship with your partner start to decrease early in the illness; work on this.

- Develop some new recreational activities such as: music, painting, scrapbooks, and collecting or even backyard golf/putting.

- Join a support group.

Tips for the Caregiver

- Be cheerful and optimistic.

- Try to keep life as normal and active as possible but recognize that you may have to adjust your living style to allow enough time for the patient's activities. Parkinson's causes slowness.

- Recognize that the patient's problems are real and may frequently change from hour to hour. The frequent changes are part of Parkinson's and its drug treatment and managing this is very demanding on you.

- Put yourself in the patient's position for a better understanding.

- Poor memory and confusion are often part of the disability and are made worse by many anti-parkinsonian and other drugs. Discuss them with your treatment team, improvement can often be made.

- Past emotional problems and anxieties may become worse.

- Counseling and emotional care are available.

- Depression occurs in 40% of parkinsonian patients.

- "You look great" or "you look better today" is very inspiring and believable from someone close.

- Denying the illness and its severity is an important method for the patient to cope with Parkinson's.

- You will be better and more able to cope if you have some help in the home and if your loved one has some time in respite care. Holidays for the caregiver are encouraged.

- Make use of the facilities in the community including Home Care, meals on wheels, visiting nurses and transportation services. Note other suggestions at the start of this section.

- The caregiver must remember to keep time aside for themselves. Develop outside interests and hobbies.

- Seek help and support from friends and family.

- Plan time together on a mutual activity you both enjoy like the theatre or walks.

- Plan ahead both in the short and long term.

- Attending support groups may help to discuss common problems and feeling with others who are in the same circumstances. It is also a good place to meet new friends with similar interests and activities.

- Go with the patient for medical and other appointments. This can be a great way to gain information, express your concerns and make treatment suggestions. However, do not speak for the patient, if the patients are able to communicate on their own.

- Make sure that you as the caregiver goes to your own doctor for regular check-ups.

- Make your problems, concerns and coping difficulties known to your treatment team. You are the person that keeps it all going and you need and deserve thoughtful compassionate considerations of your health and well being.

Both patients and caregivers (including physicians and nurses) should be careful that the lesser, and easily passed over, nuisance problems of Parkinson's are attended to. **Something positive and helpful should come out of every physician or clinic visit and this "doing something" approach can be a great comfort and morale booster for the patient**. Patients will do better and be more comfortable with their illness if they have hope. **The best strategies to enhance hope are**: the relationship between the patient and treatment team is a partnership; there is open sharing of information; and the emphasis is on potential rather than on limitations. **The patient will greatly benefit if each visit gives them feelings of**: concern, warmth and caring; problems have been listened to; the treatment plan is clear; and help and advice are available.

Care at the End of Life

A comfortable dignified death is a goal that we all wish and deserve. There are a number of facts that the patient and family should be aware of that will make this difficult time easier. It is most important that patients discuss their wishes for final care with their family and personal physician and a **living will** or **advanced** directive should be prepared. This is especially important if the situation arises where a person is helpless and unaware. The cause of this is commonly related to some other illness (for example a stroke) in addition to Parkinson's.

Caregivers, substitute decision-makers and patients need support, advice, time and attention during this most stressful and vulnerable time. Tube feeding is a major decision that arises in this situation and good information will help. There is no strong evidence that this prolongs life or prevents lung infections and it certainly does not add to patient comfort. More alert patients may just need increased assistance at meals. Ethical care of the dying patient should be directed at comfort, relieving symptoms and respecting the patient's wishes. The aim is not to hasten death. Sedatives and pain medication should be used to completely control symptoms such as severe breathing difficulty, pain or agitated delirium. Studies have shown that these drugs do not depress respiration and that patients die from their underlying disease and not from sedation given for comfort.

The withdrawal of artificial nutrition and hydration (IV fluids) is sometimes indicated and it is ethical and appropriate. It has been shown that patients can be very comfortable. Thirst is rare and is relieved with sips of fluid, lip swabs and ice chips, and restlessness and pain are controlled with morphine and sedatives. Many institutions have specially trained physicians and nurses (palliative care team) to guide and assist you. Ask for help.

Conclusion

This book has described your first step, knowing the nature and scope of Parkinson's. It then sets out the second step, the treatments and therapies available to assist in dealing with this chronic, but very treatable illness. The third step is perhaps the most important for you. It sets out what you; assisted by family, friends, treatment team and support agencies, can do to help yourself. A patient's independence and the ability to exercise some control over activities, is an extremely valuable asset not only to the patient, but also to those around them. This is attainable and this book has described how to go about achieving it; One Step At A Time.

Index

A

Acupuncture, 83
Adrenal to Brain Implants, 84
Agitation, 102
Akathisia, 44
Alcohol, 168
Alpha-Methyldopa, 21
Alpha-Synuclein, 10,11,82
Alprostadil and Muse, 117
Alternative Therapies, 67
Alzheimer's Disease, 91
Amantadine, 56,81
Amiodarone, 20
Amlodipine, 19
Anticholinergics, 58,198
Anxiety, 100,101
Apomorphine, 78,199
Apoptosis, 9,80
Assistive Devices, 210
Atypical Parkinsonism, 21

B

Bathing Aids, 180
Bathroom Aids, 211
Bedroom Aids, 212
Benserazide, 31,137
Benztropine, 59,60
Bladder Problems, 111
Bradykinesia, 2
Brain Scans, 15
Brain Tissue Donation, 87
Breast Feeding, 204
Budipine, 81

C

Calcium Channel Blockers, 19
Cane (Measuring Correct Height), 173
Carbidopa, 31,32,137
Care at the End of Life, 222
Carotid Body Cell Transplantation, 84
Catechol-O-Methyl Transferase, 51
Caudate, 8
Cause of Parkinson's, 7,77
Cell Culture Implantation, 85
Cerebellum, 15,178
Ceruloplasmin, 25
Chronic Illness, 214
Clebopride, 19
Clinical Trials, 66
Clozapine, 45,97
Cognitive Impairment, 90
Computerized Tomography, 15
COMT, 51
Conclusion, 223
Confusion and Hallucinations, 94
Confusion in Hospital, 198
Constipation, 137
Coping with Parkinson's, 214
  Tips for the Caregiver, 219
  Tips for the Patient, 217
Copper Metabolism. See Wilson's
Disease
Corticobasal Degeneration, 24
Cramps, 109
Cytosine Arabinoside, 21

D

Datatop Study, 55
Day Hospital Programs, 207
Daytime Sleepiness, 48,105
Deep Brain Stimulation, 73
Delerium, 89,90
Dementia, 89,90
Demerol, 20,54,198
Dental Care, 127
Depakene, 20
Deprenyl, 53,137
Depression & Drug Treatments, 100,101
Devices (Assistive), 210
Diffuse Lewy Body Disease, 91
Digestive System, 123
Dilantin, 21
Diltiazem, 19
Disability, 86
Domperidone, 60
Dopamine, 8,45
Dopamine Agonists, 45
Dopamine Neurons, 8
Dressing, 210
Driving, 166
Drooling, 125
Drug Adjustments, Long Term, 63
Drug Therapies, Parkinson's, 27
Drugs for Essential Tremor, 61
Dry Mouth, 57,60,126
Dying (Care at the End of Life), 222
Dysarthria, 148
Dyskinesias, 5,41
Dysphagia, 129
Dystonia, 41,42,43

E

Early Symptoms, 26,160
Eating Aids, 212
Edema (Leg Swelling), 161
Electrical Stimulation, 73
Electro-Convulsive Therapy, 101
Employment, 201
Entacapone, 51,52
Environmental Toxin Exposure, 12
Estrogen, 202
Exercise, 183
Eye Problems, 164

F

Falls, 177
Fatigue, 110
Fluctuations (Daily Mobility), 35
Flunarizine (Cinnarizine), 19
Foot (Pain and Care), 156
Fractures, 146
Freezing, 25,170
Frontotemporal Dementia, 92

G

Gait, 169
Gastric Emptying, 134
Gene Therapy, 79
Genetics, 9,11
Ginkgo Biloba, 68
Globus Pallidus, 8,69,72
Glutamate Antagonists, 57,81
Growth Factors, 82

H

Hallucinations, 94
Hoehn and Yahr, 4
Home Care and Home Making, 207
Hospital Care, 197
Human Fetal Tissue Transplantation, 84
Humour, 200
Hydrocephalus, 15,26

I

Incidence and Prognosis, 6
Insomnia, 103
Internal tremor, 160
Involuntary Movements, 41

L

Leg Cramps, 109
Leg Swelling (Edema), 161
Lesioning Procedures, 71
Levodopa, 29
Levodopa Ethylester, 32,135
Lewy body, 11,91
Lithium, 43
Low Protein Diet, 142
Lysoganglioside, 79

M

Magnetic Resonance Imaging, 15
Malignant Hyperthermia-Like
   Illness, 200
Manipidine, 19
MAO-B (Monoamine Oxidase-B), 53

Meals on Wheels, 207
Medication
   Record Keeping (Appendix), 231
   Schedule, 232
   Tips For, 63
Melatonin, 68
Memory Disorders, 89
Memory Loss (Tips For), 93
Meperidine, 20,54,198
Methionine, 79
Metoclopramide, 19,199
Monoamine Oxidase-B (MOA-B), 53,137
Motilium (Domperidone), 60
Mouth Care, 126
MPTP, 12,13
Multiple System Atrophy, 23

N

Nausea and Vomiting (Drug Related),136
Neuroleptics, 19,92
Neuroprotection, 80
Nifedipine, 19
NMDA Receptors, 45,81
Nurr1, 83
Nutrition, 142

O

Olanzapine, 97
Ondansetron, 98,200
On-Off Phenomenon, 36
Osteoporosis, 146,184
Over the Counter Drug Warning, 66
Oxidation of Dopamine, 80

P

Pain, 158
Pallidotomy, 72
Panic Attacks, 100,101
Parkinson, James, 1
Parkinson's Plus, 21
Parkinson's Society of
Ottawa-Carleton, 209
Parkinsonism (types of), 16
Parkinson's, 1
Parkinson's Associations, 209
Patient Services, 206
PET Scan, 15
Physiotherapy, 183-197
Pig Fetal Tissue Transplantation, 85
Placebo Response, 67
Placement, 208
Positron Emission Tomography, 15
Post Traumatic Parkinsonism, 25
Postural Hypotension, 118
Postural Instability, 3
Pregnancy, 203
Primidone, 18,61
Progressive Supranuclear Palsy, 23
Prolopa (Madopar), 33
Propranolol, 18,61
Prozac, 20
Putamen, 8

Q

Quality of Life, 215
Quetiapine (Seroquel), 98

R

Record of Treatment (Appendix), 231
Research and New Therapies, 77
Respite Care Programs, 208
Resting Tremor, 1
Restless Leg Syndrome, 108
Rigidity, 2
Rimantadine, 81
Risperidone, 97

S

Scales for Rating Disability, 4
Schwab and England Scale, 5
Scoliosis, 195
Selective Serotonin Reuptake
Inhibitors, 20,101,116
Selegiline, 27,53
Senior Citizen Resources, 210
Sensory Symptoms, 158
Seroquel (Quetiapine), 98
Sexual Problems, 114
Shortness of Breath, 163
Shoulder Pain, 161
Sildenafil (Viagra), 117
Sinemet (Levodopa), 27-35
Single Photon Emission Computed
Tomography (SPECT Scan), 15
Skin, 152
Sleep Problems, 102
Smell and Taste, 128
Smoking, 13
Speech, 148

St.John's Wort, 68
Stem Cells, 81
Stereotactic Surgical Techniques, 69
Stimulation, Deep Brain, 73
Striatonigral Degeneration, 24
Subthalamic Nucleus, 8,69,74,75
Surgery
  Candidates, 75
  Complications, 73
  Current Treatments, 69
  Hospital Care, 198
Swallowing Difficulty, 129
Sweating, 155
Swelling (Leg), 161
Symptoms of Parkinson's, 1

T
Tardive Dyskinesia, 21
Taste and Smell, 128
Thalamic stimulation, 73
Thalamotomy, 71,72
Thalamus, 8,69,71,72,75
Tissue Implantation, 84
Tolcapone, 51,52
Tranquilizers, 101,102,110
Transcranial Magnetic
  Stimulation (TMS), 83
Transcyclopropine, 80
Transplant-Implant Surgeries, 84
Transportation Services, 208
Travel, 213

Tremor, 1
Trihexyphenidyl, 59,60
Tyrosine Hydroxylase, 79

U
UPDRS (Scales for Rating Disability), 4

V
Valproate, 20
Vascular Parkinsonism, 25
Verapamil, 19
Viagra (Sildenafil), 117
Vincristine, 21
Visual and Eye Problems, 164
Vitamin E, 55
Vomiting (Drug Related), 136

W
Weight Loss, 142
Wilson's Disease, 25

Y
Young-Onset Parkinson's, 13

Z
Zofran, 98,200

Appendix

Record of Personal Parkinson's History and Treatment

As patients read through the book they may wish to make notes on this page about their own conditions and note page numbers that deal with their specific problems.

Patient's Name:———————————————————————

First symptoms:———————————————————————

Date diagnosed: ———————————————————————

Drug Therapy for Parkinson's:

Name of Drug   Date Started   Date Stopped   Side Effects

1. ————————————————————————————

2. ————————————————————————————

3. ————————————————————————————

4. ————————————————————————————

5. ————————————————————————————

Complications of Parkinson's and treatments:

———————————————————————————————

———————————————————————————————

———————————————————————————————

———————————————————————————————

———————————————————————————————

———————————————————————————————

Other major health problems and drugs used:

_____

_____

_____

Allergies: _____

_____

Model of a personal medication schedule
(List all drugs and keep up to date on a separate sheet and take for each visit):

Name of Drug Strength	Tablet or capsule and Amount of Drug Per Dose	Administration Times		
Example:		7am	12n	5pm
1. Sinemet	100/25	1	1	1
2.				
3.				
4.				

List questions for the Doctor on a separate sheet for each visit.

_____

_____

_____

_____

Notes

Notes